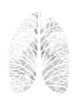

BIOENHANCEMENT TECHNOLOGIES AND THE VULNERABLE BODY

A THEOLOGICAL ENGAGEMENT

DEVAN STAHL
EDITOR

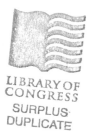

BAYLOR UNIVERSITY PRESS

Cover and book design by *the*BookDesigners
Book design by Ely Encarnación
Book design: Shutterstock/denisik11, Dychek Marina, ConnectVector

Library of Congress Cataloging-in-Publication Data

Names: Stahl, Devan, editor.
Title: Bioenhancement technologies and the vulnerable body : a theological
    engagement / Devan Stahl.
Description: Waco : Baylor University Press, 2023. | Includes index. |
    Summary: "Examines the promises and perils of bioenhancement
    technologies for those most vulnerable to health disparities: persons
    with disabilities, racial and ethnic minorities, and women"-- Provided
    by publisher.
Identifiers: LCCN 2023026712 (print) | LCCN 2023026713 (ebook) | ISBN
    9781481318273 (paperback) | ISBN 9781481318297 (adobe pdf) | ISBN
    9781481318280 (epub)
Subjects: LCSH: Transhumanism. | Transhumanism--Religious
    aspects--Christianity. | Theological anthropology. | Medicine--Religious
    aspects--Christianity. | Performance technology.
Classification: LCC B842.5 .B56 2023 (print) | LCC B842.5 (ebook) | DDC
    144--dc23/eng/20230906
LC record available at https://lccn.loc.gov/2023026712
LC ebook record available at https://lccn.loc.gov/2023026713

CONTENTS

Acknowledgments   v

Contributors   vii

Introduction   1
Devan Stahl and Adam Pryor

I Creaturely Ontology

1   **Fleshly Transhumanism**   19
*A Positive Account of Body Modification
and Body Enhancement*
Adam Pryor

2   **The Groaning of Creation**   45
Technological Interventions in Creaturely Suffering
J. Jeanine Thweatt

3   **The Tree of Life**   61
Aquinas, Disability, and Transhumanism
Miguel J. Romero and Jason T. Eberl

4   **Ontology: Where It Comes in and How It Matters**   85
A Conversation between Friends
Jonathan Tran and Jeffrey P. Bishop

II Transfiguring Vulnerability

5   **Transfiguring the Vulnerability of Suffering**   109
Kimbell Kornu

6 **This Is My Body** 133
Faith Communities as Sites of Transfiguring
Vulnerability
Wylin D. Wilson

7 **The Lame to Walk and the Deaf Fear** 151
Why It Pays for Surveillance Capitalism
to Exploit the Disabled
Brian Brock

8 **Christian Transhumanism in Context** 185
The Relevance of Race
Terri Laws

9 **Disability Justice, Bioenhancement, and the**
Eschatological Imagination 205
Devan Stahl

Epilogue 233
Enhancing Bodies: From What to What?
John Swinton

ACKNOWLEDGMENTS

This book was made possible by a generous grant from the Issachar Fund. I am indebted to Adam Pryor for helping to organize the in-person gathering that brought the grant participants together. I am also grateful to my graduate student Daniel Crouch, who helped to support the meeting and provide feedback to authors.

CONTRIBUTORS

JEFFREY P. BISHOP is Professor of Philosophy and Theology, Tenet Endowed Chair in Bioethics, Albert Gnaegi Center for Health Care Ethics, Saint Louis University.

BRIAN BROCK is Professor of Moral and Practical Theology, School of Divinity, History and Philosophy, University of Aberdeen.

JASON T. EBERL is Hubert Mäder Chair in Health Care Ethics, Professor of Health Care Ethics and Philosophy, and Director of the Albert Gnaegi Center for Health Care Ethics, Saint Louis University.

KIMBELL KORNU is Provost's Professor of Bioethics, Theology, and Christian Formation, Thomas F. Frist, Jr. College of Medicine, School of Theology and Christian Ministry, Belmont University.

TERRI LAWS is Associate Professor of African and African American Studies, University of Michigan–Dearborn.

ADAM PRYOR is Professor of Religion, Provost for Academic and Student Affairs, Bethany College.

MIGUEL J. ROMERO is Associate Professor of Health Care Ethics and Theology, Albert Gnaegi Center for Health Care Ethics, Saint Louis University.

DEVAN STAHL is Associate Professor of Bioethics and Religion, Department of Religion, Baylor University.

JOHN SWINTON is Professor in Practical Theology and Pastoral Care, School of Divinity, History, Philosophy and Art History, King's College, University of Aberdeen.

J. JEANINE THWEATT is Academic Advisor, Instructor in Philosophy and Religion, Flagler College.

JONATHAN TRAN is Associate Professor for Theology in Great Texts, Associate Dean for Faculty of the Honors College, Baylor University.

WYLIN D. WILSON is Assistant Professor of Theological Ethics, Duke Divinity School.

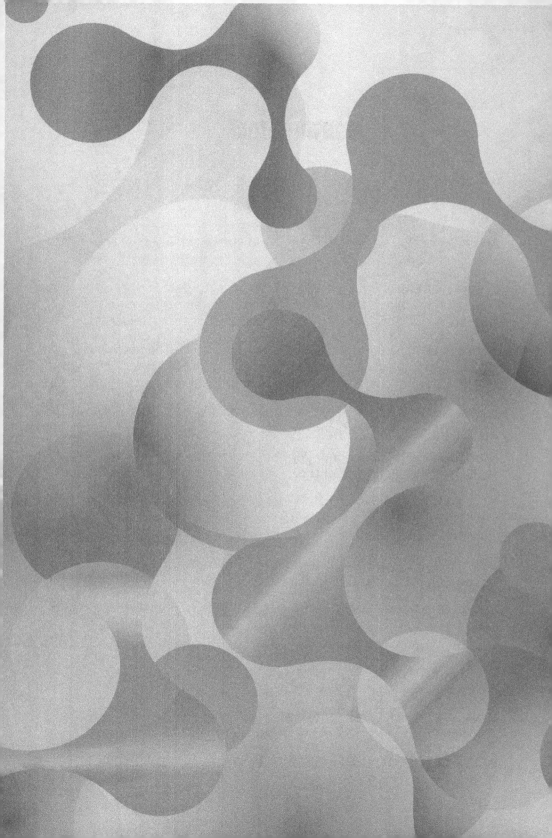

INTRODUCTION

Devan Stahl and Adam Pryor

The field of biomedical technology has experienced rapid growth in recent years. Investments in genetics, neuroscience, and psycho-pharmacology have produced revolutionary technologies such as CRISPR, brain stimulation devices, and eugeroics, which promise to treat and prevent various human maladies. Increasingly, however, these technologies (and many others) have the potential to *enhance* normal human functioning. Enhancement takes us well beyond what is merely necessary for recovery, restoration, or the sustenance of health. Within bioethics, the possibilities of enhancement have raised considerable debate.

It is notoriously difficult to find a clear line between therapeutics and enhancement—in part because it is difficult to agree upon what "normal human functioning" entails. Without a clear sense of what this norm entails, ascertaining which technologies push us beyond our natural limitations as a species is difficult. Even if a working definition of "normal human functioning" can be established for a group, the permanence, invasiveness, and capacity of specific technologies shift our perspective on what sorts of enhancements ought to be permissible.

Moreover, while there are many borderline cases, many bioen-hancement advocates see little reason to maintain a strict separation between therapeutics and enhancement. For these advocates, the goal of technological progress is not merely to restore humans to normal health but to radically exceed our natural limitations. Many bioenhancement enthusiasts, including transhumanists, believe that enhancement technologies are not only morally permissible but desirable: bioenhancement technologies will transform society for the better. With the goals of "overcoming ageing, cognitive shortcomings, involuntary suffering, and our confinement to planet Earth,"[1] transhumanists seek to radically redefine health as well as what it means to be a human person.

Both in theory and in practice, bioenhancement technologies strike at the heart of bioethical inquiry. Human enhancement raises fundamental questions about the purposes of the body as well as the goals of medicine. What are our human bodies for? Should we understand human bodies to be infinitely manipulable? Should the goal of medicine be, as the bioethicists at the Hastings Center have suggested, the prevention of disease, the maintenance of health, the relief of pain and suffering caused by maladies, the care and cure of maladies, and the avoidance of premature death?[2] Can medicine be all of these at once, or must some goals be elevated over others? Should we seek to expand our notions of "health" and "malady" and attempt to overcome limitations not directly caused by maladies? Not only should we, but do we, have a moral imperative to expand our notions of "health" and "malady"? Should we seek to overcome death itself? These questions, and the many others that have inspired this volume, press on the boundaries of how we understand human bodies and the care we offer for those bodies.

If this series of questions seems alarmist, consider this: in practice, enhancement technologies such as cosmetic plastic surgery to improve appearance, hormone treatments to improve athletic performance, and other off-label uses of drugs to increase mental stamina and alertness abound. The use of these procedures and medications remains controversial, even if they have become more commonplace. Is it not unreasonable to imagine a potentially parallel course in which one day soon what are now seen as more radical bioenhancements may also become commonplace?

Moreover, if one assumes that the development of these more radical bioenhancement technologies remains generations away, we would do well to remember that considerable investments are now being made in the areas of physical and cognitive enhancements as well as radical age extension. Some of the richest and most influential men in the world—such as Larry Ellison (CEO of Oracle Corporation), Peter Thiel (cofounder of PayPal), and Sergey Brin (cofounder of Google)—are financing research that promises to radically extend the human life span and eliminate death. That the public faces and investors in bioenhancement tend to be white, wealthy, educated men who see death as the next arena for technology to conquer should not be overlooked.

ENHANCING WHO FOR WHAT?

Given the financial investments in enhancement technology and the fundamental questions they raise about embodiment and the ends of human life, it is no wonder that Christian theologians and ethicists have become increasingly interested in these technologies. Theological anthropology has much to say about what constitutes the human as well as the moral meanings of bodily limitation and finitude. Additionally, the inherent ethical questions that accompany bioenhancement enthusiasts' promises of human flourishing and their goal of overcoming death provide a fecund space for Christian ethicists to address the vexing challenges posed by human enhancement.

Among those within the transhumanism movement, however, the more careful challenges raised by theologians are often ignored. Instead, prominent transhumanists tell a simple story about the intersection of religion and human enhancement: religious adherents are standing in the way of bioenhancement advocates by questioning whether death ought to be overcome using technology. Religious believers are sometimes derided by transhumanists as promoting a backward "deathist culture" that is preventing humans from making the world a better place.[3]

Transhumanists are perhaps right to worry that religious adherents may be more skeptical of their ultimate ambitions than nonbelievers. A 2018 national survey showed that Christians (particularly evangelicals) are less likely to agree to the use of certain bioenhancement technologies, such as those to radically improve eyesight, than nonbelievers (55 percent vs. 67 percent).[4] Other national surveys have shown that U.S. adults with high religious commitments are more likely than others to say that enhancements meddle with nature in a negative way.[5] It would appear that those who are religious are more wary of enhancement technologies and that the strength of one's religiosity may indicate a greater degree of caution when it comes to the use of enhancement technologies.

Given the skepticism many religious people have concerning enhancement technologies, one might expect that the guidance of religious leaders in confronting these technologies would be prized. However, it is increasingly clear that religious adherents no longer believe religious leaders ought to be the spokespersons for the morality of medical technologies. According to the Pew Research Center, Americans are much more likely to trust "ethics professionals" to regulate enhancement technologies than religious leaders (42 percent vs. 10 percent).[6] In fact, among the ten options for who should make decisions about the use of human enhancement technologies, religious leaders ranked last, behind the general public, government researchers, and private companies.[7]

Theological bioethicists, therefore, are in a unique position. Being able to understand the fears of the religious as well as the ethical nuances of enhancement technologies, they are a robust conversation partner for any interdisciplinary examination of human enhancement technologies that seeks to move beyond accusations that religious adherents are simply "deathists." As ethics experts (medical professionals, clinical ethicists, or specialists in topics of bioethics and technology), many of the scholars who contributed to this volume may be granted a certain amount of public trust when it comes to understanding and communicating the ethical challenges present within enhancement technologies that religious leaders appear to be lacking.

Of course, theological bioethicists are not a homogenous group. This final point is, perhaps, obvious but important. Not all of those working in theological bioethics agree on the ethics of enhancement technologies, even if they share a religious tradition. Even Christian bioethicists are diverse; they do not necessarily agree on what it means to be a human person and what it means to flourish. While the Christian tradition has had much to say about who counts as a person and our obligations toward persons, that reflection has hardly led to consensus. Yet, the theological bioethicists who are part of this volume all agree that questions of ontology, creatureliness, and personhood cannot be ignored when addressing the ethics of enhancement technologies. The judgements we make about these substantive concerns shape how we articulate the problems and potentialities that bioenhancement makes possible. How we frame creatureliness is a precursor to the ways we might form moral judgements and ethical guidance concerning human enhancement.

Certainly, in practice, general accounts of human personhood appear inadequate to provide a foundationalist grounding for a robust ethical analysis of bioenhancement technologies. Nonetheless, since human enhancements are likely to fundamentally change the ways we interact with the world around us, taking ontological, epistemological, and methodological inventory of the significance of those changes will be an ongoing task for theological bioethicists addressing these technologies. Moreover, if we do not all agree on what constitutes personhood, then it is by no means obvious that we all mean the same thing when we subsequently laud "flourishing" as a standard by which to judge ethical human enhancement. What constitutes the flourishing of human beings for some might undercut the dignity and personhood of others, an issue that is further complicated by addressing social justice questions related to whose flourishing is being assured through biomedical enhancements.

With these debates in mind, the present volume seeks to analyze the nuances of bioenhancement from the perspective of those who are often marginalized in bioethical discussions. As many liberation, black, feminist, womanist, and disability theologians have made clear, Christian conceptions of personhood have varied widely throughout history and have often been invoked to make moral and ethical judgments about specific groups of marginalized persons, typically to their detriment. The experiences of minority populations are rarely centralized in discussions concerning personhood, much less in discussions of bioenhancements. Yet, in a world of finite biomedical resources, enhancing the ability of some to flourish may hinder the flourishing of others. Unequal access to biomedical enhancements could lead to unjust conditions for people who are unwilling or unable to enhance themselves. It remains unclear what equal access to enhancements might entail and how we might alleviate inequalities that might arise.

Social justice concerns related to the use of human enhancement and access to these technologies remain woefully underthematized in Christian ethics and theological discourse. This is perhaps because those writing about enhancement, not to mention the biggest proponents of enhancement technologies, have a privileged status in our society. Those who inhabit bodies that are "othered" are often skeptical of the aims of bioenhancement technologies as well as the ambitions of transhumanists.

And of course, there is good reason to be skeptical. Historically and at present, there are well-documented inequalities in medicine that produce vast healthcare disparities in developed Western nations. From the involuntary sterilization of persons with disabilities during the eugenics movement to the decades of deceptive clinical trials on African Americans, biomedical technologies often advance on the backs of minority groups while disproportionately advantaging majority groups. Why should bioenhancements be any different? Moreover, the central premise of transhumanism is questionable from the vantage point of many minorities. Those of us with disabilities, for example, may rankle at the idea that our bodies are not only deficient but would not be optimal even if they were normalized to the current standards of health. The goalposts for what constitutes a well-functioning or flourishing body are becoming ever out of reach. Now, more than ever, there is a need for Christians to engage in thoughtful deliberation about the potentialities and challenges of technologies that seek to overcome our human vulnerabilities and finitude.

SETTING THE STAGE

In 2019, a group of twelve scholars working at the intersections of Christian ethics, biotechnology, and medicine met in San Diego as part of an Issachar Fund grant to discuss the ethics of bioenhancement technologies on minority populations. Each scholar is a member of, or works with, minoritized communities, including persons with disabilities and persons of color. The goal of the meeting was to examine the moral status of bioenhancement technologies from the perspective of these populations. The group was tasked with developing models for evaluating the

potential for human flourishing offered by various bioenhancements for those least likely to have immediate access to them.

During their first meeting, the group developed a set of consensus guidelines to direct their thinking and discussions on
bioenhancement technologies. The group used a process known
as the nominal group technique to aid them in this work. Each
member came to the meeting with a prewritten set of propositions concerning how Christians should evaluate the moral use of
biotechnologies. Every group member was given an opportunity to
share and explain the significance of the propositions they developed. As the propositions were presented to the group by their
respective authors, the facilitators began grouping these propositions into preliminary themes for further discussion.

After this initial round of presenting propositions, the twelve
scholars divided into smaller groups based on interest and research
specialties to rank the significance of the propositions and to begin
the arduous process of crafting and refining language that could be
agreed to in such an ecumenical setting. While the end product of
the process was establishing the set of twenty-five propositions in
Table 1 that were subsequently used by each scholar when writing
their respective chapters for this book, it was the discussion leading
to the formation of these propositions that was vital. The scholars
began with very different assumptions about how to characterize
the problems posed by bioenhancement. Features of their own area
of research training and theological suppositions of their Christian
community colored the original propositions each scholar developed.
By sharing our diverse understanding of ideas, refining language to be
maximally inclusive, and prioritizing shared values, members of the
group were able to generate propositions as well as common themes
that help to tie various propositions together.

The propositions developed by this group are organized into five
themes, but two larger groupings of ideas can be identified. Propositions 1–9 have a problem-and-response format. These propositions identify key issues raised by human enhancement with
significant ramifications for Christian communities, while offering
guidance that *any* adequate Christian response to these challenges
will need to address.

The concerns that the group of twelve scholars identify draw attention to the challenge of thematizing the significance of finitude, relationship, ontology, and a conception of the common good. When prioritizing vulnerable bodies, especially as this theme is developed in disability theology, these four concepts provide an essential framing for discussion of bioenhancement. An examination of human enhancement and the Christian tradition that focuses entirely on relationship but loses sight of the significance of human finitude will be incomplete. An account of the ontological significance of human enhancement that excludes questions of how our conception of the common good shapes our sense of what constitutes meaningful being will be equally inadequate. The first nine propositions provide rules of the playing field for concerns and Christian responses that a robust Christian theological or ethical account of human enhancement will inevitably need to consider.

Propositions 10–25 have a slightly different character. They become significantly more specific and focus on how conceptualizing human creatureliness allows us to embody Christ and maximally form relationship in imitation of God's grace. Here, issues of nature, malleability, poiesis, deification, perfection, and loving-kindness all take center stage. These issues provide the grist for the reflections offered in the chapters of this volume. These final propositions provide an account of Christian resources that can be theologically and ethically marshalled to respond to the challenges posed by human enhancement technologies; they also offer direction for future scholars formulating an explicitly Christian response to the use of bioenhancement technologies.

The group of scholars that formed these propositions were pluralistic in outlook; they had different concerns that emerged from the way the consensus guidelines were articulated. They continue to differ in their reading of the significance and interpretation of these propositions. As such, these propositions are not shared as though they form a foundation upon which subsequent reflection can take place. They are a tentative and shaky ground: a postfoundationalist approach to articulating how a conception of common goods and common concerns can emerge. They provide a space around which diverse theologians, with concerns and questions that might not otherwise ever overlap, can frame their work addressing human enhancement to one another so that it becomes mutually more intelligible.

Table 1: Bioenhancement Propositions

Problems/Concerns	
1.	Any time a society attempts to escape death, a wide range of harms follows.
2.	Enhancement technologies that seek to overcome death overlook how finitude shapes human nature and our processes of meaning-making.
3.	Moreover, transhumanism risks atomizing human beings and the integral relationality that comprises our personhood.
4.	These problems are intensified when public discussions of enhancement technologies obscure questions of ontology and the common good.
5.	In the absence of ontology and shared values about the common good, capitalist values become the metric of the individual and social goods.
Christian Responses to Transhumanism and Bioenhancement Technologies	
6.	A faithful Christian response to transhumanism entails analysis of the values that shape our use and development of bioenhancement technologies.
7.	Christians should question *what* and *how* bioenhancement technologies aim to enhance and whether such enhancements would be intrinsically good for individuals or society.
8.	Insofar as transhumanists seek to enhance individual freedom and autonomy, Christians should explore what this will mean for those who submit to a divine force/power.
9.	When enhancements separate humans from their bodies, their communities, or their obligations to others, Christians should consider them sinful.
Ontology/Nature and Grace/Eschatology	
10.	Christianity must engage its historical rupture of nature/grace and turn back to a metaphysics grounded in the grace of creation.
11.	This includes recognizing that human nature, as it is, is good.
12.	We do not need to become something else to reflect God's goodness; humans are already created and equipped to commune with God.

13.	As such, we affirm that human creatures exist within expanding and concentric ecologies that allow us to participate with other creatures within a Trinitarian economy.
14.	To be such a creaturely entity is to have a given form that is, in certain respects, malleable.
15.	Malleability does not imply infinite plasticity.
16.	Creaturely entities have bounded capacities whose specific attributes must be affirmed before faithful manipulation of any capacity can be undertaken.

Ontology and *Techne*

17.	Human nature and human *techne* should not be set in opposition since human nature entails human *poiesis*.
18.	Faithful development and use of *techne* must respect that Christians cannot bring about the kingdom of God through their creations, even if they can proleptically signal the coming of the kingdom through their creations.
19.	Herein lies the challenge of a creaturely ontology for transhumanism: transhumanism can become a kind of auto-deification that is anti-thetical to Christian deification that culminates in the transfiguration of humans and all creation.
20.	Transhumanism is not transfiguration; nor does it necessarily partici-pate in the Christian transfiguration of creation.

Embodying Christ and Ecclesiology

21.	An essential task of the Christian life is embodying Christ.
22.	Christ embodies a model of loving-kindness that should guide the formation of health and healing, as well as any proposition about bioenhancement.
23.	The body of Christ must be the standard for understanding human perfection.
24.	What it means to embody Christ remains relevant in a world where modifications to the body and mind take place, which can change human (and machine/technological) interaction.
25.	Therefore, acts of radical hospitality, compassion, love, sacrifice, supererogatory acts, and grace offered in imitation of Christ remain important expressions of Christian identity.

CHAPTER OUTLINES

Historically, many Christian denominations have not responded quickly or critically enough to advancements in technology. Not only this, but Christians have often neglected attention to the poor, the disabled, and the disenfranchised when endorsing certain scientific programs. The premise of this volume is that centering minority perspectives will yield new insights into biomedical enhancements. To exclude such voices from consideration, even when done unintentionally, is unacceptable for any religious tradition that calls the poor, the hungry, and the sorrowful blessed. The ontological framing of this project centers the bodies of persons who are vulnerable to health disparities with the understanding that Christians live under the divine command to care for the vulnerable among us (Matt 25:40). If all human beings reflect the image of God and are connected through their Creator, then any moral assessment of technology must consider its effects on all people, particularly those who have not historically benefited equally from technological advancements. Authors within the volume critically examine assumptions about what constitutes personhood and flourishing in most discourses on bioenhancement technologies, which tend to focus solely on privileged bodies. In short, the working group will develop axioms for an "ontology of the vulnerable."

The volume is divided into two sections. Each section deals with a unique concern over bioenhancement technologies that arise for persons whose bodies are already understood to be outside the "norm." In the first section, "Creaturely Ontology," authors describe how bioenhancement technologies challenge the ways Christians understand what it means to be human. Each chapter uses distinct theological methods and ontological suppositions to both critique and construct theological reflection on the distinctiveness of human creatureliness in relation to technology, while also examining the limits on technological enhancement for creaturely being.

In chapter 1, Adam Pryor considers how to develop an ontology of the flesh to provide a ground for evaluating transhumanist approaches to body modification. Using these concepts to give an account of how the flesh extends beyond the skin of bodies, bridging without collapsing the distance between the self and technologies in the world, Pryor uses nonideal theory and the repertories of social imaginaries to clarify how to cultivate the flesh in ways that endorse some transhumanist aspirations for human enhancement while rejecting the most radical features of transhumanism.

In chapter 2, J. Jeanine Thweatt interrogates the groaning of creation and the ontology of suffering. She argues that theology and ontology must precede bioethical inquiries into which technological interventions will alleviate creaturely suffering. Using the work of Anne Conway, she argues that the ontological difference between Creator and creation and the creaturely need for cures to physical ailments provides the necessary theological grounding for considering the question of technological enhancements. Drawing on Conway's contention that the defining ontological characteristic of creatures is a mutability that allows for participation in divine goodness, Thweatt makes the case that this ontological model is inherently open to even radical possibilities of bioenhancement. Notably, both Pryor and Thweatt reposition classic Cartesian assumptions to allow for ontologies that are amenable to and even encouraging of some forms of bioenhancement.

In chapter 3, Miguel J. Romero and Jason T. Eberl offer a Roman Catholic ontology for the disabled using the insights of Thomas Aquinas. Romero and Eberl claim disability studies and transhumanism offer two competing propositions concerning the significance of human vulnerability. Each, however, falls short in providing a fulsome account of the human person. Using the insights of Thomas Aquinas, the authors argue that the Christian account of the Tree of Life can harmonize two truths about the human body supplied by many disability scholars and transhumanists: the goodness of the human body as it is and the goodness of the human body as it could be. Aquinas' understanding of our innate creaturely vulnerabilities in relation to what the authors describe as "what–we–are" and "what–we–could–be" provides a third way for Christians to understand human bodies in their current goodness as well as their ultimate perfection.

In chapter 4, Jeffrey P. Bishop and Jonathan Tran discuss the importance of ontology for establishing personhood. Both are particularly concerned with how personhood debates affect people with disabilities. Tran argues that ontological arguments are secondary to moral action, whereas Bishop thinks the relationship between ontology and moral action is closer than Tran admits, and the intimacy of that relationship is part of what grants creaturely life its moral salience. The conversation then turns to the importance of intimacy for moral life, how Christianity does or does not make good on intimacy in how it imagines the disabled, and how bioenhancement technologies can help and hinder our intimate relationships with one another.

In the second section, "Transfiguring Vulnerability," authors consider the challenges and opportunities that come from living within vulnerable bodies and what difference bioenhancement might make for our conceptions of vulnerability. With Christ as the guide for what it means to be human, authors explore the goods and perils of vulnerability as well as what it means to inhabit a vulnerable body.

In chapter 5, Kimbell Kornu, a palliative care physician, argues that the transhumanist desire to overcome finitude and suffering through bioenhancement technologies offers a competing deification through technology as opposed to grace. With his suffering patients in mind, he argues that, for Christians, the grace of deification is partly accomplished in union with Christ by way of suffering unto divine filiation, manifesting suffering as a divine way of existing. Using the writings of Maximus the Confessor, Martin Luther, and Augustine, Kornu examines the Christian understanding of deification and transhumanism's attempted exaltation of the will, its power ontology, and its failure to appreciate shared suffering. Kornu concludes that suffering is essential to transfiguration for the Christian, and this can provide hope to those ill and suffering now.

In chapter 6, Wylin D. Wilson examines how the Christian church, as an expression of Christ's body, can become a site where our human vulnerabilities can become transfigured. In her estimation, faith communities can help humanity understand the insidious effects of normalization and the lures of bioenhancement through the practical work of embodying Christ, prophetic witness, and activism. Wilson examines how our norms for human life are shaped by ability, race, class, gender, sexual orientation, and market constraints, rather than a Christian ideal of what it means to embody Christ. The danger of normalization is that the identity of vulnerable bodies and selves is defined by their relationship to culturally imposed norms. These norms tend to other and exclude certain bodies and may even incite violence toward those who do not "measure up." Faith communities minimize the effects of culturally mediated values of normativity by reinforcing the proposition that human nature is as it is and by focusing on the transfiguration of our bodies promised in Christ.

In chapter 7, Brian Brock examines a new biotechnology—the exoskeleton—as an instance of blurring the lines between therapy and enhancement. Using disabled bodies as pawns, technology companies induce the public into sympathetic attitudes toward biotechnologies that seek to alter and perhaps even dominate bodies. The dreams of transcending human finitude and vulnerability that have generated technologies such as the exoskeleton spring from transhumanist desires to remake bodies but have no sense of what it means to live with mortal bodies in the power of the resurrecting Spirit. In opposition to such ambitions, disability theologians help us to understand the importance of making peace with our finitude.

In chapter 8, Terri Laws argues that any moral examination of bioenhancement technologies should be contextual, but the context of race is often missing within transhumanist discourse. Such colorblindness leads to a lack of empathy for African Americans as well as other racial and ethnic minorities in transhumanist discourse as well as within the technologies it promotes. Laws shows how racism within scientific medicine and Christianity in the North American context have made it difficult for transhumanists, including Christian transhumanists, to appreciate racially inclusive bioenhancement technologies. Weaving together historical case studies, black woman–authored science fiction, and black theology, Laws believes there can be an authentic Christian transhumanist movement but argues that any such movement must take empathy as its central concern.

Finally, in chapter 9, Devan Stahl explores the eschatological allure of bioenhancement technologies. Stahl's chapter places bioethicists, disability and crip scholars, and Christian ethicists into conversation concerning how to frame "justice" within bioenhancement debates. Whereas bioethicists are concerned with fair distribution of bioenhancement technologies, disability and crip scholars demand that technologies meant to serve them must recognize their inherent equality and creative natures. Christian ethicists add to these conversations a compelling account of kingdom–oriented justice that includes disabled people within the body of Christ. Stahl argues that mutual dialogue between bioethicists, disability and crip scholars, and Christian ethicists can enhance conversations concerning the place of disability in our imagined futures.

What both sections make clear is that what constitutes human flourishing is an open issue in our pluralistic society. Human normalcy is not simply given. It is rooted in ontological assumptions about our creatureliness and the ways in which that creatureliness is enhanced or denigrated by its mutability. It follows, quite logically, that "enhancement" is often ambiguous. The lines between therapeutic uses of technology and technologies used for human enhancement are becoming less sharp each day. As the pace of developing new and increasingly intimate enhancement technologies quickens, the questions raised here about human normalcy and mutability will only become more salient.

While the Christian tradition has had much to say about who counts as a person and our obligations toward persons, there has been little scholarship that considers how Christians should understand enhancement technologies. Perhaps even more importantly, there has been even less consideration given to these questions from the perspective of the most vulnerable in our society. The second section of this volume begins to address this lacuna and is an invitation to future reflection. We hope that the present volume begins a wider conversation: framing the moral debates surrounding bioenhancement technologies through the lenses of marginalized perspectives, creating a more robust approach to the ethics of human enhancement.

Notes

1   Humanity+ Board, "Transhumanist Declaration," website of Humanity+, last modified March 2009, https://www.humanityplus .org/the-transhumanist-declaration.

2   Mark J. Hanson and Daniel Callahan, introduction to *The Goals of Medicine: The Forgotten Issues in Health Care Reform*, ed. Mark J. Hanson and Daniel Callahan (Washington, D.C.: Georgetown University Press, 1999), ix.

3   Zoltan Istvan, "Can Transhumanism Overcome a Widespread Deathist Culture?" *Huffington Post*, May 26, 2015, http://www.huffingtonpost .com/zoltan-istvan/can-transhumanism-overcom_b_7433108 .html.

4   Debra Whiteman, Jeff Love, G. Rainville, and Laura Skufca, "U.S. Public Opinion & Interest on Human Enhancement Technology," AARP

Research, January 2018, 17, https://www.aarp.org/content/dam/aarp/research/surveys_statistics/health/human-enhancement.doi.10.26419%252Fres.00192.001.pdf.

5   Cary Funk, Brian Kennedy, and Elizabeth P. Sciupac, "U.S. Public Wary of Biomedical Technologies to 'Enhance' Human Abilities," Pew Research Center, July 26, 2016, https://www.pewresearch.org/science/2016/07/26/u-s-public-wary-of-biomedical-technologies-to-enhance-human-abilities/.

6   Funk, Kennedy, and Sciupac, "U.S. Public Wary."

7   Funk, Kennedy, and Sciupac, "U.S. Public Wary."

I
CREATURELY ONTOLOGY

1

FLESHLY TRANSHUMANISM

*A Positive Account of Body Modification
and Body Enhancement*

Adam Pryor

"Creaturely Ontology" might seem like a strange place for a book on transhumanism to begin. After all, issues of justice, equality, and freedom all make intuitive sense in the context of considering the ethical ramifications of the issues so often associated with transhumanism, such as body modification or radical life extension. Ontology is a bird of a different feather from the more traditional values of bioethical analyses insofar as it might be used to address the complex questions raised by transhumanist aspirations.

Yet perhaps that is because ontology is a little misunderstood. Ontology deals with the "furniture of the universe." Its purview is that whole set of things that are said to exist. And while, on the face of it, what counts as existing may seem so facile and obvious as to not need to be considered when addressing transhumanist questions, I would ask that you pause a moment and suspend that judgment. Philosophically, I would ask that any reader take the time to engage in what we call a phenomenological *epoché* (a bracketing or a pause) in order to engage in the prospects of doing *transdisciplinary public theology* as a form of correlational theology:[1] linking various existential questions arising from transhumanism with theological means of making meaning of our existence.

What I intend by transdisciplinary public theology need not be the focus of this chapter, but I want to emphasize from the beginning that I assume any transdisciplinary project requires abandoning unwavering commitments to monodisciplinary constructs. To pursue the sense of social well-being that motivates transdisciplinary engagement, one must commit to a degree of disciplinary skepticism that gives space for other fields of study to enrich our accounts of these common concepts.[2] We must acknowledge the ways other fields tell us something meaningful about the world in a way that is *better* than how it could be accounted for by our own discipline—pumping the brakes on how our everyday, disciplinary-driven encounter with the world would proceed.

This process of bracketing opens the door to discovering newly meaningful constellations of being. We find, even if not permanently, new patterns for organizing existence that yield distinct, different, and sometimes conflicting accounts of who and what is due sufficient respect—who and what really count—as we mete out goods such as justice, equality, and liberty in our moral calculus. Whether we acknowledge them explicitly or uncritically adopt them, our ontological assumptions, which are so often tied to methodological and disciplinary suppositions, shape the field in which our ethical and moral dilemmas can be played out.

One could certainly still question from the outset, why do we need to begin with critically interrogating ontology? Does transhumanism really so drastically change our understanding of being that fundamental questions of ontology need to be reconsidered? Does transhumanism disrupt what counts as furniture in the universe? I will not pretend to answer that question in its entirety, here; however, the tendency in this section is to say, "Yes, it does." Different styles of theological thinking will give different reasons for the affirmative response to this question. For my part, as a correlational theologian, I would use Paul Tillich to indicate why transhumanism requires we engage with fundamental questions of ontology.

Tillich makes the case that there are five dimensions of things: inorganic, organic, psychological, spiritual, and historical. Something belongs to one of these dimensions based on the way it modifies four basic categories of ontology that he articulates in a distinctly Kantian fashion: space, time, causality, and substance.

"These categories have universal validity for everything that exists. But this does not mean that there is only *one* time, space, and so on. For the categories change their character under the predominance of each dimension. Things are not *in* time and space; rather they *have* a definite time and space."[3] Each dimension unfolds experiences of time, space, causality, and substance that modify preceding experiences of these categories in irreducible ways. In short, each dimension makes a novel way of existing in the universe possible. For correlational theologies this is important, because the existential questions shaping how theological reflection on meaningful life is pursued will be expressed differently depending on the predominant dimension adopted.

The question that correlational theologians might ask, then, is, in what ways is transhumanism modifying how our senses of time, space, causality, and substance interact such that the intersection of the existential and theological processes of meaning-making constitute a new way of being in the world? Insofar as transhumanist discourse is doing this, one would need to do the work of fundamental ontology to consider the ramifications opened by these shifts.

I and, for their part, the other authors in this section are making the case that we must critically and conscientiously define that ontological field on which our moral and ethical reasoning occurs given the radical implications of transhumanist arguments. In the context of transhumanist tendencies to escapist and elitist fantasies that can all too easily denigrate the natural limitations of bodies and the ecosystems in which those bodies thrive, accounting for creaturely ontologies becomes more important than ever. Vice versa, a ham-fisted naturalism that rejects the technological modifications and goods a carefully reasoned transhumanism might provide is equally stultifying. *Taking the time to carefully consider how we constitute meaningful units of being in the world can be a powerful precursor to making moral judgments regarding transhumanist discourse.* This is too easily glossed over in existing work at the intersection of theology and transhumanism. Moreover, this work only rarely is able to sufficiently account for the reality of vulnerable bodies that are often most intimately engaged with forms of bioenhancement.

Thus, in this chapter, I want to use features of Maurice Merleau-Ponty's phenomenology of the "flesh," Elizabeth Anderson's account of nonideal theory for addressing categorical inequality, and Charles Taylor's repertories for social imaginaries to offer an alternative ontological ground for evaluating transhumanist aspirations to body modification. In principle, this ontological grounding could be used to critique aspects of transhumanist aspirations for radical life extension as well, but I will not address that issue in depth here. I would argue that the philosophical tools enumerated above provide a better grounding for transhumanist aspirations than the typically Cartesian framework of transhumanist discourse that treats the body as a limiting factor to infinitely extending the life of the mind. Instead, combining features of these theorists' work allows for the development of flexible ontological units in which the body extends into the world around it such that the chiasmic bridging of self and world creates different fleshly boundaries from the barriers of our skin. Yet, understood in light of Anderson and Taylor, these bodily extensions are never the provenance of the individual. They occur in the context of wider social networks forming repertories for building new, more just, social imaginaries. When it is sufficiently understood that no specific iteration of the flesh is the ideal, but that each can occlude our perspective and give rise to unintended, though nevertheless real, instances of social closure and marginalization, we can begin to develop standards for cultivating the flesh in ways that neither simply reject nor wholly endorse transhumanist aspirations.

THE FLESH

An ontology that makes use of the phenomenological concept of "flesh" might help provide some preliminary answers to thinking about the way transhumanism yields ontologically significant insights on distinct existential questions that cannot be ignored by any form of correlational theology. I invoke the term "flesh" (or what has sometimes been called "flesh of the world") in the spirit that it has been used by Maurice Merleau-Ponty in his later writings: where his phenomenology proleptically invokes an indirect or elemental ontology.[4]

Briefly put, "flesh" describes how Being is always given over as a depth. This depth is indirectly communicated by the mutually institutive intra-action of beings incarnating a body and adventing the world around that body. The goal of using this philosophical concept, "flesh," was to overcome the implications of the seemingly commonsense assumptions attached to a Cartesian way of dividing up existence into subjective thinking things (*res cogitan*) and objective extended things (*res extensa*).[5] Instead, "flesh" designates an intertwining or enlacement—an *Ineinander*—by which self and world unfold together.

Thus, the flesh makes carnality axiomatic. We are characterized by our sharing in corporeality; we are a body in the midst of other bodies that comprise the flesh.[6] While it is tempting to think that this sharing in corporeality connotes that we are all simply material, physically constituted of common stuff, this would not be correct. Flesh indicates much more than some common atomic structure or existence as bare materiality; this is because flesh is not exactly "something" in a substantialist sense.[7]

Instead, the flesh is like an "element." The elemental typically designates something that cannot be well accounted for by traditional philosophy.[8] Flesh is "the formative medium of the object and the subject . . . one cannot say that it is *here* or *now* in the sense that objects are; and yet my vision does not soar over it."[9] Or, as David Macauley describes it, flesh "serves as a 'concrete emblem' of a way of being."[10] Still, this way of being that is the flesh is not a substance to itself—it does not play by the rules of existence and nothingness, nor does it emanate from an ideal form. The flesh is natal in its elementality: it gives birth to an irreducible reversibility of self and world that is transcendent of both and mutually imminent to both.[11] In this way the flesh is a distinct type of being arising from the complex entangling of our everyday sensibilities about self and world.

This element of flesh is always realized *indirectly* and manifests *between* me and the world synchronizing these disparate realities. Thus, to understand this sense of the flesh as an element, we have to consider how it is manifested through the encounter of beings, because I cannot engage the flesh except through these encounters even if it is not sufficiently characterized by any one of these particular encounters itself. As Glen Mazis rightly suggests, flesh stands between the general and the particular: a mediate—between the Being of ontology to which we are given indirect access through its happening in the contact of particular beings in the sensible world.[12] Perhaps it is best to say we catch glimpses of the flesh: not as a "something" we can directly set ourselves toward, but as the pre-reflective, abyssal grounds or insights that are realized through *but also make possible* the particular, specific sensible contact of beings.

An example is necessary to begin clarifying what is thus far an immensely technical description of the flesh.[13] I rode my bicycle to work in my office this morning. I grabbed the dropped handlebar of my road bike and felt the gritty texture of the handlebar tape under my palm. As I swung my leg over the top tube, my knee bumped into the firm nose of the saddle, sliding the whole frame a bit underneath my body, and my hand slipped onto the rubbery hood of the brake. In the space between my thumb and forefinger, I could feel the pressure of my body leaning into the hood as I tried to regain my balance to keep from falling over.

In this initial aspect of the encounter—where I feel features of the bike—there is a chiasm at work. Chiasm refers to a crossing or intersecting in the field of the flesh. More technically, the chiasm describes the encroaching of a perceptive event (e.g., my hand feeling the handlebar tape, touching the brake hood, or my knee bumping the saddle). The crossing of the chiasm does two things that we can immediately note. First, it makes me aware of the obverse quality of the body. Above I described the shared carnality of the flesh: the flesh occurs as bodies in the midst of the world that in sensing are able to be sensed. Here this sensing and being sensed is expressed as a quality of my body enacting the flesh. The lived-bodies of the flesh exhibit a *reversibility* in themselves.

Second, the crossing or intertwining of the chiasm is evocative. It is not just that my hand and the handlebar tape happen upon each other. The encounter yields a grittiness. Similarly, the brake hood that my hand slips onto gives a rubbery sensation, and the nose of the saddle offers up a resolute firmness, eventually bruising my knee. These encounters of chiasmic entwining evoke a sense that neither I nor the bicycle possess beforehand; nor is this encounter well described by some combinatorial logic (the sensibility is not something additive). A distinct way of being or quality of the world is emerging through this crossing of the flesh; as we mutually inhere to one another, a different way of being in the world begins to take shape.

The experience of reversibility is never simultaneous, though.[14] It is crucial that this experience of sensing and being sensed never collapses into an undifferentiated unity (a sensing my own sensing). The crossing of a chiasm, as with the various senses of the flesh that different configurations of my encounter with the bicycle evoke, would not be possible without a distance or separation. If I *am* the bicycle and the bicycle *is* me, there is not a sufficient sense of distinction to have a crossing. The chiasmic encounter of the flesh relies upon this difference: there remains a separation or a distance between us—what is usually called an *écart* or dehiscence.

This separation, though, is not a hard-and-fast concept sharply dividing perceiver from perceived. Such a concept would violate the carnality of the flesh and could never accommodate the evocative quality of lived-experience that the chiasm describes. Instead, the separation or distance is an opening (as is well-described by subsequent deconstructionists). It is an opening or a space between the perceiver and the perceived that makes any quality of sensibility possible. To better understand why this is not a sharp division, let us return to the encounter with the bicycle.

Having regained my composure (and giving a quick check to see if anyone has seen me nearly tumble while inflexibly getting on my bicycle), I push hard with my right foot onto the pedal. It creaks slightly against my weight, but the whole frame seems to leap forward, and the saddle settles gently underneath me. I never cease to marvel at how every downward push on the pedal seems to throw me forward on this composite frame as opposed to the mushier lurching of the first steel-framed road bike I ever owned. A few more turns and I feel the cleats on my shoes snap into the clipless pedals and my legs spin more easily and freely as the road opens onto a long downhill stretch. It is cold today, and the wind bites at my cheeks as I shift down the rear cassette so that my legs do not start spinning too fast on the pedals during the descent.

As I ride down the hill, feeling the pedals turn over under my feet, any separateness of me and the bicycle gives way to our entwining. We move around potholes opening up before us as my arms extend into the handlebars so that the bicycle is incorporated into the space of my body. My legs are not separate from the pedals anymore but become pistons that pivot on a confusion of feet and crankarms so that the bike leaps forward, as though it wants to and I am merely there to make this expression of itself possible. I experience the bicycle at different moments as separate and intertwined: distant and then inseparable from the lived-space of my body—me and then not-me.

This tension between the experience of entwining and dehiscence defies our typical understandings of self and world, but it arises by looking into the sensed depth of these evocative encounters that we are naming flesh. My riding the bicycle helps illustrate a swift movement beyond any imporous border of individuation—as though my sense of being remains strictly divided along a dermal barrier. In the intertwinings and gaps of perceptive events, there is an incarnating of the self. *I* come to be through my perceptive incorporation of the bicycle that is no longer separate from me. Grammar hardly seems to do justice to the experience this chiasmic encounter evokes: "We *is* a deft vehicle descending the hill." At the same time there is an adventing of the world in this act of incorporation—a promise of manifesting otherwise silent possibilities. Slaloming pothole obstacles and the wind biting at my cheeks are aspects of the world that could easily go unnoticed without the speed that my entwined body-bike achieves going down the hill. What develops is "a *pregnancy* of possibles, *Weltmöglichkeit.*"[15]

Yet, what of the *écart*? It cannot be left behind so that our chiasmic entwining simply becomes simultaneous; however, is that not precisely what has happened in descending the hill? While we can easily flip back and forth between sensing and being-sensed as distinguishable conditions, there is something that our perceptual experience shows to be artificial in this division. We lose something of the perceptual phenomenon if we adhere to a stark separation of divisible moments in our fleshly encounters.[16]

These divisible moments encroach upon one another so that finally the flesh evokes something distinctive—the "we is" of the body-bike—that pushes the *écart* to a new frame of reference felt at the borders of the bike tires with the road or the tingling skin of my cheeks; these two experiences are no longer so disparate as they once might have been understood to be, as if one belonged to the bicycle and the other to my body. The experience of me and the bicycle as not-me crossing in the flesh falls away here in our *availability* to one another. Instead, a newly incorporated, hybrid—even cyborg—body advents upon a world that is now felt differently; a new set of chiasmic crossings in the flesh becomes possible adventing new ways of being in and understanding the world.

With the flesh as this primordial ontological unit, we find ourselves to be in a state of flux. The shape these entanglements of the flesh may take are not permanent. After all, I eventually arrived at my office and hopped off my bike. My feet and legs no longer turn as pistons over wheels that give me felt contact with the ground. Now the weight of my body rests on my heels as I walk awkwardly over the cleats in my shoes, and it is my feet that give me a lived-experience of the ground once again. The mutability of my various folds of the flesh becomes clear. The sensibility evoked is not permanent, nor is it forever gone; the flesh is mutable—crossing and uncrossing, tangling and untangling—letting these instances of evocative encounter rise up and fall away. My senses of space, time, causality, and substance differentiate such that a real difference between my cyborg bike–body and everyday walking body opens up before me when the flesh, with its chiasmic encounters, becomes *the primordial unit of our ontological thinking.*

This indirectly revealed flesh makes for promiscuous beings:[17] beings constantly engaged in the persistent metamorphosis of incorporating and adventing made possible as instances of the flesh's noncollapsed intertwining. These promiscuous beings yield a poetic and fragile ontology. It is, to borrow the idea from Bachelard, a penumbral ontology wherein the borders of ontological units are fuzzy as they bubble up in the contexts of particular practices and modes of working in the world, only to be reshaped relationally under the guise of new contexts.[18]

Whether or not this shift constitutes a new dimension as described in terms of Tillich's work above could be debatable: one could argue the differences experienced in the ontological categories here are still compossible to one another. For a different dimension to be opened in the flesh, a greater difference in the experiences of space, time, causality, and substance would need to emerge—something, perhaps, that does not occur with my bike-body cyborg as compared to the walking body but would remain possible with the incorporation of more extensive technologies imagined by transhumanist body modification.

Yet, to dwell too long on this point is to forget this penumbral quality of the flesh as an ontological unit. It lacks the permanence that we typically associate with ontologies that frame themselves in terms of being or becoming. What is more important than deciding if shifts in the flesh are compossible to one another in terms of space, time, causality, and substance is to understand the ways in which the flesh can be constantly reshaped relationally. This fundamentally relational ontology of the flesh has limits. You cannot be whatever or whoever you want to be in the flesh. The irreducible social components that condition the relationships we can have with the world make only certain incarnations of the lived-body in the flesh available to us. Moreover, those possibilities of being enfleshed are not inherently equal.

NONIDEAL THEORY

Given this irreducible social dimension of the flesh, critical to the conception of a preliminary ontology that I am putting forward is the idea of a relational account of systematic group inequality developed by Elizabeth Anderson. Her account is explicitly a "nonideal theory." In her work *The Imperative of Integration*, Anderson considers how such a theory applies to the issue of affirmative action. Of particular concern for her, in a way that I would argue is prescient to issues in transhumanism, is the shift that occurred in late 1960s leftist political movements from "redistribution" to "recognition."

Following the work of Nancy Fraser,[19] Anderson makes the case that a shift toward identity politics laid the groundwork for an account of American multiculturalism that distracted us from addressing integration and the reality of racial inequality. She contends that without a thorough account of how segregation of social groups promotes group inequality, an undemocratic tendency toward inequality will persist. In short, even if the multiculturalist hope that recognition will lead to equality is well-intentioned, it is also fiction.[20]

It is not difficult to analogically extend this argument to transhumanism. On the one side stand the enhanced human beings with certain upgraded body modifications that give them a set of social, political, or economic advantages. On the other side stand those nonmodified human beings. Even if the nonmodified are *recognized* as deserving dignity, their *integration* to social spheres providing access to technologies that facilitate the development of valuable social capital, political influence, and class mobility can be stymied. Recognition will not automatically produce equality.

Anderson lauds nonideal theory in the face of such well-intentioned recognition for three reasons. First, it takes seriously human beings as actual human beings. We are not perfectly rational or just, and any adequate theory for addressing social ills or imagining alternative ontologies must take our deficiencies into account.

Second, nonideal theory requires us to take our problems seriously and investigate them thoroughly. Calling for robust empirical investigation of the challenges we face, Anderson contends that our ideal theories too often occlude our perspective. When adopting idealist approaches to account for systemic disadvantages, we can too readily assume that the challenge we face is rooted in a gap between reality and the ideal we envision; we rarely take sufficient time to understand if that ideal sufficiently frames the reality of the phenomena in question.

This leads directly to a third advantage of nonideal theories: they do not hide injustices the same way that ideal theories can. If we begin from an idealized perspective, we cannot give sufficient credence to the standpoints of those who are already marginalized; their marginalization can be written off as a product of the imperfect distance between reality and the ideal. Nonideal theory requires us to remain open to the counterfactual possibilities closed off by an idealist account of justice and its underlying ontology.[21]

Before following Anderson further, I want to pause and consider what this might mean in terms of transhumanist discourse and the flesh. Anderson does not have in mind an ontology of the flesh as I have described it here. Still, her account of nonideal theory is critical to the flesh. As mentioned above, not all lived-bodies can take up the flesh in the same way; social conditions affect how the world is presented to the lived-body. My example of riding a bike to work, though simple, illustrates this well. There are a variety of lived-bodies that cannot incarnate this account of the flesh because they do not have access to a bike. The phenomenological *epoché* applied to that everyday experience for me can only make sense if that everyday experience is made available to other sorts of lived-bodies. All sorts of social conditions and decisions may create systemic disadvantages to pursuing such an incarnation of the flesh. In the case of the bike, this might include things like the safety of the streets one rides on, the distance one lives from work, the requirements of hygiene when one arrives at work, or disposable income to purchase a suitable bicycle that will not break down.

This list could go on and on. If something like Anderson's approach to nonideal theory is made axiomatic to an account of the flesh, then we prevent the flesh from running headlong into the three problems outlined by Anderson with idealist approaches to addressing categorical inequalities. Vice versa, modifying Anderson's approach, by employing the flesh as an ontological unit, prevents idealizing specific ontological units. The individual alone cannot incarnate the flesh; the flesh requires an analysis of the available horizon in which the lived-body is engaged. There is a fundamental entanglement of self and world entailed by the flesh as an elemental ontology. As such, it requires robust analysis of the myriad ways the flesh emerges, and none of these incarnations of flesh can be ignored based on their proximity to an assumed ideal.

While we may not worry too much about incarnating bike-bodies in the flesh, when the kinds of incarnations of the flesh include even more significant incorporations to the lived-body as imagined by transhumanism, the stakes are raised. Incarnating the flesh of bodies with modularized bio/synthetic parts (as commended by many transhumanists) creates a more drastic categorical inequality expressed in the standpoints of populations marginalized by such technologies (Anderson's third point above) and requires a more robust analysis of whether this idealized vision of the human body sufficiently frames how we might best incarnate the flesh (Anderson's second point above).

In pursuit of this nonidealist theory, Anderson weds Charles Tilly's account of durable inequalities with Iris Young's typology of oppressive group relations.[22] The relationship between ontology and justice outlined by the work of either of these political philosophers deserves a chapter unto itself. For our purposes, let it suffice to say that *Anderson approves of Tilly's robust account of how categorical inequalities between groups are generated and sustained irrespective of the internal constitution of those groups.* Tilly adapts Weber's understanding of

social closure (where a group obtains dominant control over a potentially important good), in order to apply it to processes like opportunity hoarding (preventing other groups access to the controlled good)
and exploitation (allowing limited access that deprives an out-group
of the full productive value of their efforts to use or produce that
good) to account for how inequalities are perpetuated. Further, using
emulation (copying the inequalities of one group into the working practices of another) and adaptation (copying a norm or habit
of inequality from one domain into another), categorical inequalities
can be made systemic quite quickly.[23]

Tilly's account makes clear that inequality spreads without
regard to the intentions of individual actors, and prejudicial ideol-
ogies rationalizing inequality are contextualized in terms of social
closure. Thus, conscious prejudice is not made into an individu-
alizing cause of inequality; it is contextualized in terms of its production through the persistence of systemic group inequalities.
What Anderson rightly identifies is that segregation is the "linch-
pin of categorical inequality"[24] in Tilly's work. Specifically, "segregative processes consist of any intergroup relations (laws, norms,
practices, habits) by which one identity group closes its social
network to counterpart groups."[25] By augmenting Tilly's argument
with Young's more complete account of the causal mechanisms
of inequality (including her analyses of how violence and conquest have perpetuated categorical inequality, how the leverag-
ing of control extends categorical inequalities, how political power
institutionalizes inequality, how prejudice reproduces inequalities
underlying intergroup interactions, and how the account of labor
and production must be modified by procedural analyses), Anderson gives a more complete account of how these segregative processes take shape.[26]

With these theoretical concepts in hand, Anderson "locates the
causes of economic, political, and symbolic group inequalities in
the relations (processes of interaction) between the groups, rather
than in the internal characteristics of their members or in cultural
differences that exist independently of group interaction."[27] If the
relations between groups, rather than individual actors, are taken
as primary in pursuit of a just, democratic society, then inequalities
in the distribution of a good can be deterred, but this cannot occur
through the actions of *individuals*.

REPERTORIES AND SOCIAL IMAGINARIES

At the heart of a thorough consideration of transhumanism lies a well-known problem for political philosophy: How might we address "the persistence of large, systematic, and seemingly intractable disadvantages that track lines of group identity, along with troubling patterns of intergroup interaction that call into question our claim to be a fully democratic society of equal citizens"?[28] Anderson may be analyzing the actuality of racial grouping, but the dark side of transhumanism potentially has this same problem inchoately lurking. The question we must ask is, "How can nonideal theory be helpful in addressing segregationist inequalities as these are applied to the unrealized potentialities of transhumanist discourse?" and "What role can alternative ontologies play in creating modern social imaginaries to prevent us from perpetuating inequalities through unreflective action?"

I am certainly not using the term "modern social imaginaries" exactly as Charles Taylor might. There remains in Taylor's account a sense that social imaginaries are shared moral conceptions of the ideal society. Yet, he is clear that, different from social theory, social imaginaries describe "the ways people imagine their social existence, how they fit together with others, how things go on between them and their fellows, the expectations that are normally met, and the deeper normative notions and images that underlie these expectations."[29]

Social imaginaries are intended to bridge the gap between theories held by a minority of social elites and the assumed, common praxes underpinning social norms. Because social imaginaries deal with this common understanding and practice, Taylor intends that they be applied widely. The social imaginary is not about individual, specific societal practices. Rather, it functions much like a horizon in phenomenology: examining the factual and normative background that often remains unarticulated but informs the holistic understanding by which we incorporate and make sense of particular theories and practices.[30]

Here I invoke the concept of social imaginaries not for their idealism but for the ways that an imaginary shapes and constitutes normative notions of legitimate social existence through images and stories that respond to the perceived problems of a particular age.[31] Specifically, my interest in the social imaginary relates to the helpful concept of a repertory. A repertory is "the collective actions at the disposal of a given group of society."[32]

Repertories are critical to distinguishing social imaginaries from social theories: these are the collective sets of actions that make sense of our moral order and make the norms of the moral order realizable. Without this actionable element of a social imaginary, the imaginary would not be able to take on the quality of a horizon in its shaping our understanding of those all-too-obvious-to-mention facets of our world.[33] In the course of giving examples of the way the repertory participates in shaping our social imaginaries and transforming our society, Taylor outlines two critical principles: "(1) the actors have to know what to do, have to have practices in their repertory that put the new order into effect; and (2) the ensemble of actors have to agree on what these practices are."[34]

What I am suggesting here is that the ontologies we create are like a set of stories that give shape to the repertory of our social imaginary. The claim, at this point, is inherently neither positive nor negative. Here, then, I am imagining ontology to be a type of counterfactual imagination that at its best can legitimate all-too-hidden injustices (both real and looming on the horizon) and can help us creatively transcend the seemingly insurmountable quagmires these injustices reveal.

As our creaturely ontologies give shape to a repertory of choices we might make, what Taylor makes clear is that this repertory solidifies a meaningful order to the world. If making different ontological assumptions can yield alternative repertories of possibility for collective action, then understanding the ontological implications of transhumanism matters immensely for developing models of transfiguring vulnerability or creating wider justice, equity, and access to bioenhancing technologies. Moreover, insofar as transhumanism tends toward a dualistic, ontological idealism that reinforces a segregating inequality, applying Anderson's approach to nonideal theory can provide a crucial corrective to the typical transhumanist repertory in which recognition of differences does not lead to resisting the systemic production of inequalities.

THE HUMAN BODY 2.0

How then do we bring together these threads from a phenomenology of the flesh, nonideal theory, and repertories of social imaginaries as they apply to features of transhumanism? How do we talk about effective body modifications in this ontological flesh? Are all body modifications acceptable, or are only some means of modifying the body to take up the flesh acceptable? And why is modularized bio-enhancement in an ontology of the flesh different from modularization understood from a more typical Cartesian dualism?

As a test case, I want to consider the work in the *H+Pedia* on the "Human Body 2.0."[35] The material in this introduction is facile. Still, it provides a helpful introduction to philosophical assumptions being made in transhumanism. Moreover, it invites us to imagine how those philosophical assumptions could be amended such that the bodily enhancements envisioned can be grounded with philosophical nuance in order to remain sensitive to issues such as the vulnerability of bodies, concerns of justice, and concerns of equity.

This particular model of thinking about transhumanism, from the "Human Body 2.0," relies heavily on thinking about how hybrid, bio/synthetic structures could be used to create modular means of repairing or augmenting human bodies. The analogy that is drawn on extensively compares and contrasts the human body to a car:

> One of the big differences between, say, a car and a human body is that you can easily remove a part from a car and replace it with another part *without having to damage the car*. Suppose that the human body could be designed from the ground up to be more like a car, in the sense of being able to remove and replace faulty parts without major trauma? Diseased and damaged tissues and organs could be swapped for healthy ones (assuming replacements were available, which is a separate matter) without surgery, without pain, quickly, safely and without any need for a healing process afterward.[36]

Driving this car analogy further, the authors of this page of *H+Pedia* suggest:

> This approach would mean that any disease or damage to the organs could be quickly and effectively dealt with (i.e., eliminated entirely) by replacing the affected parts with new, healthy ones, just like you would remove and replace a faulty or worn-out air filter in a car. There would be no danger of infection during the process because the biological part would be safely inside its

module the whole time, so bacteria, viruses etc., would have no access to any living tissue, even when the body was wide open to the outside world.[37]

The elements of treating the human body as a machine or substrate on which the human mind serves as a model of personhood are clear in a quote like the one above. It implies an allusion to a loose Cartesian ideology. However, the philosophical allusion can be made far more specific. Descartes' *Treatise of Man* outlines developmental processes that could, hypothetically, be isolated and then used as models for medical intervention and bodily repair exactly akin to changing out worn-down parts from a machine.[38]

Still, the ontological approach I have outlined here is actually more amenable to this car analogy than one might suppose at first, though for wholly non-Cartesian reasons. The hope of having modular organs or bodily enhancements that can be attached and then removed from the body as situations arise is not all that different from my account of riding a bicycle wherein the feeling of the world extends into the handlebar and wheels of the bicycle. The vision of transhumanism integrates these technologies more intimately, *but the modularity imagined is not inherently problematic.*

Using the flesh, as an ontological model, however, would entail that there is no ghost in this hybrid technological machine. There is no mind or spirit that might be utterly separated from the modular lived-body. As such, we might look to effective phenomenological accounts of disability theory as providing us some crucial caveats for describing effective and just body modification. The analysis of lived-experiences of persons with disabilities offered by Nancy Eiesland in her now classic work *The Disabled God* continues to stand the test of time in many ways. Other, more contemporary accounts could certainly be invoked here, but by building on Rebecca Chopp's critical praxis correlation, Eiesland develops a model for deconstructing the naturalization of the body that is well suited to the transdisciplinary public theology I described at the beginning of the chapter.

Eiesland narrates how the lived-experience of the hybridity of disabled bodies opens onto an "emancipatory transformation" whereby the mutability of the body is revealed through newly realized freedoms stemming from the incorporation of insensate technologies. She carefully illustrates how the specificity of the technological embodiment pursued matters (there is no one-size-fits-all account of how body modification is universally positive or negative) and how the social accomplishment of any biomodification or bioenhancement is critical to the lived-experience of augmenting the body.[39] Further, the incorporation of any technology modifying the body cannot be passively assumed; the technology has to be understood as an active contributor to a new sense of embodiment (a new shaping of the flesh) that is not merely additive (a body plus a technology) but transformative (a new type of hybrid body).[40]

Imagine for a moment, then, *any* technology added to the body, enhancing its function. Where that technology opens emancipatory transformations and is transformative of the body itself in crucial ways, that body modification can be thought of as an enfolding of the flesh. The work of transhumanism is then, philosophically speaking, *likened to a host of innocuous uses of technologies for modifying bodies.* As I write this chapter, I am using my reading glasses to see the words of the notes I made more clearly. The glasses are not merely a passive addition to my body but transform the clarity with which I see the notes and the speed with which I can work. They extend my vision and would hardly be controversial as a form of body enhancement. Philosophically, I am suggesting we argue that my use of reading glasses or riding a bicycle can be thought of as analogous to more radical transhumanist bioenhancements like modifying limbs or organs. These bodily enhancements may be radically different in the degree of modification, but they are not fundamentally different in kind.

Making this analogy relies on two assumptions, though. The first assumption is that the implicit tendency toward a Cartesian separation of mind and body has to be utterly abandoned. Cartesian dualism makes the body into a passive technology inhabited by the mind. The body sits in the same inert, ontological category as all the technologies being appended to the body on this metaphysical framework. The body and its appended technologies are like Lego bricks being put together: purely additive and never transformative.

In a Cartesian framework, the extension of sensation of the body into the bicycle that I described in the flesh simply *could not* occur.

My description of feeling the road through the wheel of my bicycle would be a nifty psychological projection in a dualist framework, not an ontological reality as I have suggested. Instead, if the body is the mutable site of the mutual constitution of self and world in the flesh, then the way the body takes up technologies is a transformation of flesh otherwise unrealizable apart from the specificity of the technology incorporated. The body and the technological bioenhancement are active partners forming a peculiar way of instantiating the flesh and thereby navigating our experience of self and world. No matter how in-depth or superficial the bioenhancement might be, its ontological status in relation to the body is always made "active" in its formation of flesh.

The second assumption is that the technology that enhances or modifies the body has to be recognizable as part of a repertory of an available social imaginary. The radical aims of transhumanist body modification push up against this boundary. Understanding body modifications as philosophically analogous to more innocuous versions of incorporating technology to the flesh creates an avenue for expanding the repertories of our social imaginaries. In short, talking about transhumanist body modifications as parallel to everyday technologies (bicycles, reading glasses, etc.) tells a story about body modification that resists essentializing, normative accounts of what kind of body is morally and socially acceptable. Too often this liberating potentiality in transhumanist discourse is lost because it too readily adopts a Cartesian denigration of the body that is philosophically unnecessary at best and highly problematic at worst.

What remains problematic in a project like "Human Body 2.0" is the ambiguity of the ideas presented. If we take up the notion of the flesh with the caveats provided by nonideal theory, then the spitballing speculation of transhumanists, as with a page like the "Human Body 2.0," is highly problematic. Anderson is clear that any sufficient ontology is going to need to accept the foibles of our humanness, investigate the problems we confront in a specific and thorough way, and take seriously the perspective of the marginalized. Vague analogies that treat the human body like a car hardly suffice. Even if the ontological possibilities opened by thinking of all technological bioenhancement and body modification in terms of the flesh as being similar in kind but not degree are reasonable, it is only through expanding the repertories of our social imaginaries that specific instantiations of this flesh can become socially acceptable; *and* that cannot occur without the careful attention to the problems and pitfalls of using *specific* technologies for *particular* bioenhancements.

When we look more closely at particular project pages in the "Human Body 2.0" project, though, we can begin to imagine just how complex this issue becomes. To close, I want to develop a little thought experiment. I want to extrapolate ontological implications, with the help of some science–fiction imagining from one cited project in the "Human Body 2.0," related to organ building, that focuses on the ability to create 3–D shapes from living tissue.

Citing a 2017 study on the ability to grow tissues in vitro that mimic structural motifs of corresponding tissues in vivo, the "Human Body 2.0" project makes extensive use of how "an engineering framework for guiding autonomous tissue folding" could then be used to create complex 3–D structures.[41] This approach, which has more recently been incorporated into approaches to bioprinting that rely on cellular morphogenesis, has vast potential applications: from studying tissue development and repair to disease modeling. As advances in lithography bioprinting and spheroid bioprinting continue, organoid engineering that can model and produce complex 3–D tissue structures is rapidly becoming less and less of a science fiction.[42] How modular these tissues would be (as is an assumption with the transhumanist example comparing the body to a car with parts that could be replaced) is still highly questionable. However, the potential to create alternative tissue structures that could be incorporated to lived–bodies is becoming more possible than anyone might have imagined even a few decades ago.

Organoid engineering and bioprinting provides a model for creating significant, malleable, and intimate bioenhancements through tissue repair and modification. Imagine, for a moment, this technology is used to develop enhanced lung tissues that prevent miners from suffering from various forms of pneumoconiosis (diseases like "black lung"). Through bioprinting, the shapes of specific lung tissues could be manipulated to prevent the impregnation of fine dusts that come to destroy otherwise healthy tissue. Essentially, by manipulating the shapes these tissues take, miners could have a built-in sieve that prevents or severely limits the likelihood of developing chronic disease later in life.

Providing bioenhancements to miners based on these technologies could easily be imagined in terms of taking up new ontological assemblages of the flesh that would be positively received in the repertories of existing social imaginaries (i.e., providing miners a modified lung tissue that prevents debilitating future disease seems just). This initial positive reception could then be further evaluated based on the ways that these means of taking up flesh (ontologically speaking) would or would not establish categorical inequalities for in-groups (enhanced lung-tissue recipients) and out-groups (non-enhanced lung-tissue recipients). If bioprinting tissues that created new ensembles of the flesh entailed forms of social closure through exploitation (only allowing coal miners, not silicate miners, access to the newest shapes for tissue printing) or opportunity hoarding (preventing particular groups of miners from getting access to these bioenhanced tissues at all), then this ontological avenue becomes inherently unjust through the social segregation it would entail. The place of this formulation of the flesh in the repertories of our social imaginaries could change quickly and dramatically.

What is curious about this little thought experiment is how closely it ties the ontological to the ethical. Even if a particular form of bioenhancement opens onto new means of shaping the flesh, the place of these ontological possibilities in our repertories of social imaginaries conditions the way these formulations of the flesh can be experienced. Anderson's approach to nonideal theory complicates our ontology. The ethical and moral valuations of categorical inequalities that may be created by or develop out of these instantiations of the flesh cannot be neatly separated from these formulations of the flesh in themselves. I would never suggest that this chapter has disentangled the thorny issues that arise at this intersection of ontology and ethics in my particular reading of transhumanist bioenhancement. However, perhaps I have at least convinced the reader a bit more than when we began that beginning with a consideration of our creaturely ontologies is essential if we want to take transhumanist aspirations seriously in all their most admirable and terrifying possibility.

Ontology and ethics are constantly intertwining on this model. And it is perhaps this oscillation between ethics and ontology that is most significant theologically. In a Christian theological framework that takes this ontological flesh seriously, our ethical sensibilities about justice, equality, and grace should constantly be directing the ways we enfold the flesh of the world. This is not to say a static prospect of the kingdom of God serves as an ideal toward which all ways of taking up the flesh should be directed. Instead, it is to claim that we must be always attentive to *all* the ways our bioenhancements (from bicycles to bioprinting tissues) form repertories of social imaginaries that promote the flourishing of God's kingdom.

It is for this reason that I believe bioenhancement propositions 17–20 outlined in the introduction of this book are so critical to this chapter or *any* Christian account of transhumanism. Human nature entails *poiesis*. The project of what it means to be human and to flourish is ongoing and flexible. The way we incarnate flesh is never static. Thus, it requires a constant attention to the ways in which our poietic possibilities are working in tandem with the proleptic possibilities of God's care for creation, while never suggesting that our powers of bioenhancement might lead to the idolatrous idea of auto-deification or some form of soteriological transfiguration. If we respect that the transfiguring power of God lies beyond the capacities of bioenhancement and that the mysterious possibilities of the transfiguration of creation are not a simple ideal onto which our ontological imaginations must be fixed, then we are freed to enrich the flesh in creative ways. We are freed to imagine new ways human *techne* can steward the ontological possibilities of God's good creation.

NOTES

1   For a more robust description of this method, see Adam Pryor, *Living with Tiny Aliens* (New York: Fordham University Press, 2020).

2   Robin W. Lovin, Peter Danchin, Agustín Fuentes, Friederike Nüssel, and Stephen Pope, "Introduction: Theology as Interdisciplinary Inquiry—The Virtues of Humility and Hope," in *Theology as Interdisciplinary Inquiry: Learning with and from the Natural and Human Sciences*, ed. Robin W. Lovin and Joshua Mauldin (Grand Rapids: Eerdmans, 2017), xxiii–xxiv.

3   Paul Tillich, *Systematic Theology* (Chicago: University of Chicago, 1951–1963), 3:18 (emphasis original).

4   Lawrence Hass persuasively makes the case that there are three interrelated senses in which Merleau-Ponty uses the term "flesh" that need to be kept in mind and distinct when reading his work. See Hass, *Merleau-Ponty's Philosophy* (Bloomington: Indiana University Press, 2008); and Adam Pryor, *Body of Christ Incarnate for You* (Lanham, Md.: Lexington, 2017), chap. 5. Here I am eliding features of the three senses of flesh to focus on the constructive potential of what Hass identifies as the least developed facet: flesh as an elemental ontology.

5   See also Adam Pryor, *The God Who Lives: Investigating the Emergence of Life and the Doctrine of God* (Eugene, Ore.: Pickwick, 2014); and Pryor, *Body*. Some of what appears here can also be found formulated with different emphases in those works.

6   Hass, *Merleau-Ponty's Philosophy*, 138.

7   For Merleau-Ponty what is common is a certain "style" of being—a form of expressive movement (most evident in perception) that characterizes the way in which different body-schemas make space for one another in the midst of the flesh (i.e., shared corporeality). On style see Maurice Merleau-Ponty, *Phenomenology of Perception*, trans. Colin Smith (New York: Routledge & Kegan Paul, 1962), 378ff.; Merleau-Ponty, *Signs*, trans. Richard C. McCleary (Evanston, Ill.: Northwestern University Press, 1964), 112ff.; and Scott L. Marratto, *The Intercorporeal Self: Merleau-Ponty on Subjectivity* (Albany: SUNY Press, 2012), 101–4 and 157–59.

8   See also Richard Kearney, *Anatheism: Returning to God after God* (New York: Columbia University Press, 2010), 89–90.

9   Maurice Merleau-Ponty, *The Visible and the Invisible*, ed. Claude Lefort, trans. Alphonso Lingis (Evanston, Ill.: Northwestern University Press, 1968), 147 (emphasis original).

10   David Macauley, *Elemental Philosophy: Earth, Air, Fire, and Water as Environmental Ideas* (Albany: SUNY Press, 2010), 308; citing Merleau-Ponty, *Visible and the Invisible*, 147.

11   Merleau-Ponty, *Visible and the Invisible*, 148–49.

12   Glen A. Mazis, *Merleau-Ponty and the Face of the World: Silence, Ethics, Imagination, and Poetic Ontology* (Albany: SUNY Press, 2016), 265–66. This is not simply testifying to the long-held supposition that Being is only actualized through beings that are never in turn precisely equivalent to Being. Flesh is manifest in the contact *between* beings and the world. Flesh belongs not to *a* particular being but to an encounter.

13   See the examples in Merleau-Ponty, *Phenomenology of Perception*, 140–45; and *Visible and the Invisible*, 147–48. I am taking these as the impetus for my own example of riding a bike.

14   Merleau-Ponty, *Visible and the Invisible*, 133. On this separation see also Mazis, *Merleau-Ponty*, 60–62; and Jean-Paul Sartre, *Being and Nothingness*, trans. Hazel E. Barnes, reprint ed. (New York: Washington Square Press, 1993), pt. 3, chap. 2.

15   Merleau-Ponty, *Visible and the Invisible*, 250 (emphasis original).

16   Hass, *Merleau-Ponty's Philosophy*, 128.

17   On the promiscuity of being see Pryor, *Body*, chap. 8.

18   Mazis, *Merleau-Ponty*, 266–67.

19   See Nancy Fraser, "From Redistribution to Recognition? Dilemmas of Justice in a 'Postsocialist' Age," in *Justice Interruptus* (New York: Routledge, 1997), 11–39.

20   Elizabeth Anderson, *The Imperative of Integration* (Princeton: Princeton University Press, 2010), 1–2.

21   Anderson, *Imperative of Integration*, 4–7.

22   See Charles Tilly, *Durable Inequality* (Berkeley: University of California Press, 1999); Tilly, *Identities, Boundaries, and Social Ties* (New York: Routledge, 2016); and Iris Young, *Justice and the Politics of Difference* (Princeton: Princeton University Press, 1990).

23   Tilly, *Identities*, chaps. 5–8 and 10.

24   Anderson, *Imperative of Integration*, 9.

25   Anderson, *Imperative of Integration*, 9.

26   Anderson, *Imperative of Integration*, 8–14.

27   Anderson, *Imperative of Integration*, 16.

28   Anderson, *Imperative of Integration*, 3.

29   Charles Taylor, *Modern Social Imaginaries* (Durham, N.C.: Duke University Press Books, 2003), 23; Taylor, *A Secular Age*, 1st ed. (Cambridge, Mass.: Belknap Press of Harvard University Press, 2007), chap. 4.

30   Taylor, *Modern Social Imaginaries*, 24–25. Taylor uses the idea of social imaginaries to trace the divergence of multiple modernities; in particular, he traces the expansion, embedding, and shifts in the concept of moral order that is critical to understanding Western modernity and corresponding senses of self-identity that arise. See Charles Taylor, *Sources of the Self: The Making of the Modern Identity*, reprint ed. (Cambridge, Mass.: Harvard University Press, 1992), chap. 1.

31   Taylor, *Modern Social Imaginaries*, 23ff.

32   Taylor, *Modern Social Imaginaries*, 25.

33   Taylor, *Modern Social Imaginaries*, 28–29.

34   Taylor, *Modern Social Imaginaries*, 115.

35   "Human Body 2.0," entry in *H+Pedia*, April 30, 2020, https://hpluspedia .org/wiki/Human_Body_2.0.

36   "Human Body 2.0" (emphasis original).

37   "Human Body 2.0."

38   René Descartes, *Treatise of Man*, trans. Thomas Steele Hall, Harvard Monographs in the History of Science (Cambridge, Mass.: Harvard University Press, 1972).

39   Nancy L. Eiesland, *The Disabled God: Toward a Liberatory Theology of Disability* (Nashville: Abingdon, 1994), 22–42.

40   Sharon V. Betcher, *Spirit and the Politics of Disablement* (Minneapolis: Fortress, 2007), 94–99.

41   Alex J. Hughes et al., "Engineered Tissue Folding by Mechanical Compaction of the Mesenchyme," *Developmental Cell* 44, no. 2 (2018): 165–78, https://doi.org/10.1016/j.devcel.2017.12.004.

42   Andrew C. Daly et al., "Bioprinting for the Biologist," *Cell* 184, no. 1 (2021): 18–32, https://doi.org/10.1016/j.cell.2020.12.002; Ozan Erol et al., "Transformer Hydrogels: A Review," *Advanced Materials Technologies* 4, no. 4 (2019): 1900043, https://doi.org/10.1002/admt.201900043; Takanori Takebe and James M. Wells, "Organoids by Design," *Science* 364, no. 6444 (2019): 956–59, https://doi.org/10.1126/science .aaw7567; Fan Zhang and Martin W. King, "Biodegradable Polymers as the Pivotal Player in the Design of Tissue Engineering Scaffolds," *Advanced Healthcare Materials* 9, no. 13 (2020): 1901358, https://doi .org/10.1002/adhm.201901358.

2

THE GROANING OF CREATION

Technological Interventions in Creaturely Suffering

J. Jeanine Thweatt

The broad theological starting point for the following reflections is the need for discernment in answering an always pressing and urgent question: What can we say in the face of creaturely suffering? In one mode of theologizing, this gives rise to the question, "How can this be?" and, thus, to the project of theodicy, the impulse to justify belief in the existence of a definitively good Creator God despite the demonstrable fact of evils and the suffering they cause. In another mode of theologizing, this gives rise to a more practical question, "What shall we do?" and, thus, to the project of compassion, the impulse to render aid to the sufferer.

It is this mode of theologizing that interests us when we ask questions about technologies of human enhancement; even in the more extreme futurist, imaginative depictions of enhancements as positive augmentation of existing capacities, or the enabling of entirely new capacities, the meaning of such interventions depends upon the implicitly understood context of the limitations and vulnerabilities of present human embodiment. While this context is not identical to the state of being we might call active suffering, it includes the possibility of it, and perhaps even the inevitability of it. So, the question of technological enhancement is always a question of intervention in the possibility of suffering.

This may sound like we are gearing up to move straight into the realm of the ethical, but, at this point, I want to turn us back to the theological—not to ask the straightforward theodicy question, but to ask a theological and ontological question hiding behind it, a question about the nature of Creation, or what it means to be a Creature. To put it bluntly: Is suffering a part of what it must mean to be created, to be a creature?

To consider this question, I will use the work of Anne Conway, who provides an intriguing entry point into questions about the nature of God and of Creature, the relationship of Body and Spirit, and the reality and purpose of creaturely suffering.

WHY ANNE CONWAY?

A preliminary word of explanation is in order for the choice of a figure hailing from the seventeenth century as the major theological voice on a topic usually addressed in a strictly contemporary, even futurist, orientation. What can a seventeenth-century thinker, however genius or prescient, have to say about the issues of human technological enhancement that concern us here—moreover, a figure who, until very recently, has remained entirely obscure and absent from the received Western philosophical and theological tradition?

One simple reason to choose Conway is the contribution such a choice represents to the larger historical and philosophical project of recovery of such voices. As Sarah Hutton observes, in Conway's *Principles*, we have "the fullest and most systematic work of philosophy by any woman writing in the English language in the seventeenth century."[1] And, yet, with Conway living at a time when only a minority of women were formally educated and philosophy was viewed as an exclusively male endeavor, her exceptional position as a woman recognized widely in her own time as an able philosopher was ultimately not enough to keep her from historical obscurity. It is only recently that recognition of her work and place in the Western philosophical tradition has begun to be acknowledged.[2]

Simply contributing to the recovery of this philosophical and theological voice is, however, insufficient as a reason for the employment of Conway here. The decisive factor in this choice reverses the emphasis of the inevitable and skeptical question above. Choosing a historical figure so distant from the questions of human enhancement that we are theologically confronting underscores an important point: the questions we confront are not "new," in the sense that they are unprecedented, or unique to our age. Rather, these questions are the contemporary forms of questions that were being confronted in the seventeenth century no less urgently than we confront them now, in our own millennium. While the occasion of these confrontations changes from age to age, the substance of them remains consistent: What do these technologies show us about who we are? What do these technologies make possible, and what should we do with these possibilities?

Moreover, the contemporary forms of these questions (Should we seek to become "better than well"? Should we participate in the quest for radical life extension?) are what they are *because of* the historical legacy of seventeenth-century issues. The dualistic, mechanistic view of matter and the view of nature as an exploitable resource given to human dominion continue to persist in the Western philosophical and theological tradition and undergird projects like those promoted in the transhumanist movement. Conway's challenge of these assumptions in conversation with the thinkers who constructed and promoted them demonstrate that these are not self-evident or necessary assumptions and that contemporary critique is not unprecedented.

Finally, Conway confronts these questions from a position that is grounded in an immediate experience of bodily vulnerability and suffering. She constructs an explicitly theological ontological system of the "Creature" that takes this ever-present possibility into account—while simultaneously exploring, in her personal life, the cutting-edge technological (medical) interventions available to her from the leading philosophers, scientists, and physicians of her day. Thus, in Conway, we have a thinker who is both an innovative philosopher and an ardent Christian believer seeking understanding of her own situation. While constructing a theological system mapping the categories of Being, she is navigating the questions of the actuality and necessity of creaturely suffering, both theologically and personally. The result is a nuanced theological position, which recognizes the reality of creaturely suffering, while making space for the attempt to alleviate that suffering and for the potential trans-formation of the creature.

READING THE *PRINCIPLES*

In encountering Conway's text, it is helpful to keep in mind the following: the fragmentary nature of the work, the eclectic theological nature of the work, and the broad philosophical context of the work.

As noted above, Conway's place in the Western philosophical tradition is a matter of ongoing recovery and is not necessarily simple. In part, this is the result of the paucity of material; we have only the one publication to reflect a lifetime of philosophical and theological reflection. Further, this comes to us as an anonymous and posthumous publication, primarily through the efforts of Conway's friend and physician, Francis Mercury van Helmont. The *Principles* are described in a prefacing note, "To the Reader," in the original publication as composed "for her own use, but in a very dull and small character; which being found after her Death is partly transcribed (for the rest could scarcely be read)."[3] Later, van Helmont describes them as "broken fragments," which were "abruptly and scatteredly, I may also add obscurely, written in a Paper Book, with a Black–lead Pen, towards the latter end of her long and tedious Pains and Sickness, which she never had Opportunity to revise, correct, or perfect."[4] This description underscores the importance of reading Conway's work as a sketch—a series of notes-to-self meant to catch the outlines of an original and inventive comprehensive metaphysical system.

It is also the case that Conway's text can strike the beginning reader as an idiosyncratic, eclectic metaphysical system that draws its inspiration from the various and seemingly arbitrary resources and materials available to Conway in the form of friends, acquaintances, and works of contemporary medicine, philosophy, and theology. Hutton notes that her "incorporation of religious and theological material in her treatise, in particular her use of kabbalistic and Origenist doctrine, runs counter to our sense of the modernity of seventeenth-century philosophy, and even our idea of philosophy."[5] Conway's late conversion to Quakerism is also evident in the *Principles*, particularly in its influence upon her theology with regard to suffering.[6]

The *Principles*, as its lengthy subtitle suggests (see foot-note), addresses one of the most urgent questions of the day, the relationship between spirit and matter.[7] Conway situates her phil-osophical system as not simply a refutation of Cartesian dualism but a system that solves a set of interrelated difficulties generated by the separate philosophical proposals of Descartes, Hobbes, and Spinoza. This philosophical context provides an insight into why Conway conceptualizes substances in the way that she does; her ontology, at least in part, is a creative solution to the central prob-lem of Cartesian dualism.

Conway was also deeply influenced by the Cambridge Pla-tonists, through her brother and her friend and admirer Henry More. The Neoplatonic character of her thought can be seen, for example, in the way her doctrine of Creation is reminiscent of a doctrine of emanation, and in her concept of an ontological Ladder of Being, with all creatures oriented toward the Good.

CONWAY'S TRIPARTITE THEOLOGICAL ONTOLOGY

Conway begins with a consideration of the nature of God. From this starting point, Conway derives the rest of her metaphysical categories. There are three categories of beings that exist: God, Christ, and everything else, which she calls "Creature."

Conway's theological starting point is not substantially different from classical theism: "God is a Spirit, Light, and Life, infinitely Wise, Good, Just, Mighty, Omniscient, Omnipresent, Omnipotent, Creator and Maker of all things visible and invisible."[8] In this first section of Chapter 1, we hear echoes of both the Platonic concept of the divine and the Nicene Creed. In section 4, Conway draws the conclusion that "in [God] there is no Time, nor any Mutability," and it is this characteristic of divine immutability, connected to her understand-ing of eternality, that is the crucial ontological distinction between God the Creator and God's creatures.[9]

This leaves Conway with the same theological problem that any classical theist inherits, and she solves it in much the same way. A God who is immutable and eternal is necessarily, by that nature, separate from the ever-changing, time-bound realm of existence of God's creation. How can such a God create? How can such a God relate to Creatures? This dilemma is addressed by the existence of

Christ, who is the Middle nature and Mediator, partaking of aspects of both God and Creature, enabling a relationship that does not conceptually endanger the ontological boundaries envisioned.[10]

The category of Creature, then, quite literally encompasses everything else in creation: "Creature, or whole Creation, is but one Substance or Essence in *Specie*, although it comprehends many individuals placed in their subordinate *Species* and indeed in Manner, but not in Substance or Essence distinct from one another."[11] The boundaries are defined by the nature of beings with respect to mutability; Conway writes, "Here is therefore a threefold Classis or rank of Beings: The First whereof is that which is wholly unchangeable: the Second changeable only to Good; so that that which in its own Nature is Good, may become yet better: The Third is that which though it was in its own Nature indeed Good; yet could be indifferently changed, as well into Good, as from Good into Evil."[12] To be Creature, then, is to be something whose defining essence is that it can be transformed for either better or worse.

It is the final category of Creature that concerns us the most. What does it mean to be Creature? What does it mean for mutability to be the defining aspect of Creature, and what does this suggest for how we think of ourselves within it? Conway's consideration of this ontological category and its relation to the other categories of Being (God and Christ) leads us to three key areas relevant to our current inquiry: the concepts of spirit and matter, mutability and perfectibility, and the role of physical suffering.

CONWAY'S "MONISTIC VITALISM"

Jane Duran describes Conway as a "monistic vitalist who sees the world as composed of an intriguing mixture of spirit and matter."[13] Reading Conway's work as primarily a response to Cartesian dualism, she writes, "A great deal of what philosophically motivates Anne Conway is the desire to expose the falsity of the bare, mechanistic account of the universe, of emerging views of nature as inert, dead substance, with which she (and others who were aware and literate at the time) was becoming increasingly familiar."[14] This motivation is most clearly visible in the final chapter of the *Principles*, which bluntly declares, "The Philosophers (so called) of all sects have generally laid an ill Foundation to their philosophy, and therefore the whole Structure must needs fall"—the so-called philosophers in question being Descartes, Hobbes, and Spinoza.[15] Conway herself describes her philosophical system here as "being so far from Cartesian . . . that it may be truly said it is Anti-Cartesian."[16]

Conway's critique of Cartesian dualism resembles that of another recently recovered female philosophical voice of the time, Elisabeth of Bohemia, whose personal correspondence with Descartes contains the devastating question, "How can the soul of a man determine the spirits of his body so as to produce voluntary actions if the soul is only a thinking substance?"[17] Conway's version of this question is, "If Spirit and Body are so contrary to one another, so that a Spirit is only Life, or a living and sensible Substance, but a body a certain Mass merely dead . . . What (I pray you) is that which doth so join or unite them together?"[18]

Unlike Elisabeth, whose only extant philosophical work is her correspondence, Conway offers in the *Principles* not simply a critical question but a sustained attempt to offer a solution through the construction of a comprehensive ontological system. Conway solves the problem of how spirit may animate "dead matter" by proposing that there is no such thing as "dead matter"—rather, all that exists, as Creature, is a mixture of spirit and matter, and these interpenetrate and interact in all things. Duran summarizes the reasoning thus: "The argument . . . is that, since it would be impossible for 'dead matter' to give rise to motion, it is necessary to hypothesize that from the beginning of the material world, gradations of spirit were already found in all existent things."[19]

MUTABILITY AND TRANSFORMATION

For Conway, the essential, defining ontological characteristic of Creatures is mutability; to be a Creature is to be the kind of thing that inevitably changes over time. Her consideration of the implications of this defining characteristic takes the form of follow-up questions: How much can Creatures change, in what ways can Creatures change, and for what purpose?

Conway first considers "whether one Individual can be changed into another of the same or a different Species." To this, she answers no, on the basis that "for then, the very Essences of Things would be changed," adding that this would "make a great confusion," and would be contrary to the Wisdom of God—without individual identity, she writes, we would exist in a world of such instability that knowledge and truth itself would be impossible.[20]

Second, she asks "whether one Species of Things can be changed into another." By "species," here, she means something like the common meaning of natural kinds, rather than her own categories: "For the *Species* of Things are nothing else but Individuals digested, or comprehended, under one general *Idea* of the Mind, or common Term of speaking."[21] Her answer is that there may be apparent change, but not essential change: "One Species essentially or substantially distinct from another, cannot be changed into another, even as one Individual cannot be changed into another." She concludes by observing that if Man is a "species" and Horse is a separate "species," then "if *Alexander* cannot be changed into *Darius*, he cannot be changed into his own Horse *Bucephalus*."[22]

The reasoning here, however, rests primarily on the previous argument regarding the necessity of individual identity and is not an argument for the stability of the concept of natural kinds, which is helpful to keep in mind as Conway returns to her threefold ontology. "In order to know how far the Mutations of Things can reach, we must examine how many *Species* of Things there be, which as to be Substance or Essence are distinct from one another," Conway writes, concluding that, properly speaking (as opposed to the sloppy, common use of the term "species"), "we shall find only Three."[23] The resulting conclusion is that Creatures cannot transform into God or Christ, for this would be an essential change; but Creatures, as individual members of one substantial category, may indeed mutate in ways that stretch the common-usage meaning of the term "species."

The point of this, for Conway, is not simply that Creatures are mutable but that Creatures, through their mutability, are intended to participate in Divine Goodness. The potential for transformation is simultaneously ontological and moral. Philosophical systems that multiply ontological categories and define essences according to natural kinds make a fatal mistake in her judgment: "For so every Creature is so exceedingly straitly bounded, and strictly included and imprisoned within the narrow limits of its own *Species*, that the Mutability of Creatures is wholly taken away: Neither can any Creature variously exercise any greater participation of Divine Goodness, or be advanced or promoted to any farther perfection."[24] This is further clarified in the following example:

> First, let us take an Horse, which is a Creature indued with divers degrees of perfection by his Creator, as not only strength of Body, but (as I may so say) a certain kind of knowledge, how he ought to serve his Master, and moreover also Love, Fear, Courage, Memory, and divers other Qualities which are in Man: which also we may observe in a Dog, and many other Animals: Seeing therefore the Divine Power, Goodness, and Wisdom, hath created every Creature good; and indeed so, that it might by continual augmentations (in its Mutability) be advanced to a greater degree of Goodness, ad infinitum, whereby the Glory of those Attributes do more and more shine forth. . . . Now I demand, whether the Spirit of an Horse hath in it such infinite perfection, that a Horse may always become better and better *ad infinitum*, and yet so as to remain a Horse? . . . Again, I ask whether the Species of Creatures do so infinitely one excel another, that an Individual of one particular Species may still go forward in perfection, and approach nearer unto another *Species*, but yet never reach so far as to be changed into that *Species*? As for instance: An Horse in divers Qualities and Perfections draws near unto the Nature and Species of a Man, and that more than many other Creatures; Is therefore the nature of a Man distant from the Nature of an Horse, by Infinite Degrees, or by Finite only? If by Finite, then certainly a Horse may in length of Time be in some measure changed into a Man, (I mean his Spirit; as for his Body that is a thing evident).[25]

Conway concludes this rumination by suggesting that we should conceptualize the relationship between the different varieties of Creature as proximate steps on an infinite Ladder, stretching endlessly toward perfect goodness, and that individuals may progress from one step to another, without ever crossing the ontological boundary that separates Creator from Creature.[26]

THE ROLE OF SUFFERING

Despite the clear Neoplatonic influences evident in her system, Conway's ontology creatively and deliberately resists the kind of negative conception of matter as inherently recalcitrant to the spiritual. In rebuffing Cartesian dualism in the way that she does, Conway also conceives of creaturely existence as material–spiritual, opening the possibility of a theological consideration of bodily experience that, though not always positive or pleasurable, is always purposeful. This allows Conway to see the role of suffering as central to the moral progress and transformation of the creature.

Conway bases her theology of suffering on the foundational notion of creaturely mutability: every Creature is on a path of transformation, either drawing closer to God or falling away from God. But, drawing upon a concept of Evil as privation, she posits that while it is possible to pursue Good ad infinitum, it is not possible to pursue Evil infinitely, for there is no such thing as infinite Evil. Instead, a creature who "degenerates," or falls away from the Good, experiences the consequences commensurate to its action.[27] It is the specific experience of pain that provides the creature motivation to return to its proper pursuit of the Good, not as a response of fear to further suffering or divine punishment but through a stimulation of the element of Spirit or Life itself, which is inseparably part of every living creature: "Every Pain and Torment excites or stirs up an operating Spirit and Life in every thing which suffers, as we observe by continued Experience, and Reason teacheth us, that of necessity it must be so; because through Pain, and the enduring thereof, every kind of crassitude or grossness in Spirit or Body is attenuated . . . and so the Spirit . . . is set at Liberty, and made more Spiritual . . . through suffering."[28]

She follows this disciplinary theodicy logic to its conclusion, in a doctrine of universal redemption, writing, "Hence it may be inferred, that all the Creatures of God, which heretofore degenerated and fell from their primitive Goodness, must after certain periods be converted and restored, not only to as good, but unto a better State than that was in which they were created: For Divine Operation cannot cease: . . . it uncontestably follows, that it must at length return unto Good; and by how much the greater its Sufferings are, so much the sooner shall it return and be restored."[29] This view of suffering as a mechanism of universal redemption certainly owes much to the influence of Origenist thought, available to Conway through her association with the Cambridge Platonists, and brings to mind parallels with the modern "soul–making theodicy" of John Hick.[30]

However, there is more to be said with regard to Conway and the role of suffering than simply reporting on her relatively brief theological remarks. For most of her life, Conway was afflicted by debilitating illness and chronic pain, and this experience directly impinges on her philosophy.[31] In her intellectual biography of Conway, Sarah Hutton draws upon the work of physician Thomas Willis as a primary source regarding Conway's physical condition. In Willis' description, Conway began suffering recurrent headaches before the age of twelve, after her recovery from a fever, which would last for days at a time and during which she could not tolerate light, noise, speech, or movement. These episodes began to occur more frequently as she grew older, until, at the time of her consultation with Willis, she was "seldom free."[32]

Hutton suggests, "It is more than likely that her own incontrovertible experience of bodily pain affecting her mind contributes to her refutation of mind–body dualism in the passage in her *Principles* where she asks, 'Why does the spirit or soul suffer so with bodily pain? . . . If one admits that the soul is one nature and substance with the body . . . then all the abovementioned difficulties vanish.'"[33] Likewise, it seems a reasonable supposition that this personal experience influenced her theological understanding of bodily pain, serving the purpose of a purifying chastisement meant to return the creature to the Good.

Yet even this is not all that should be said, for we also know that Conway spent considerable time seeking out medical expertise and pursuing innovative treatment, even while holding a theological view of suffering as a mechanism for returning creatures to the Good. Hutton's summary of the various treatments Conway tried includes baths and spa waters, bloodletting, faith healers, a near–fatal dose of quicksilver, tobacco, coffee, a "red powder" from Wales, and a "blew powder" prescribed by a Dr. Johnson; in 1656, she traveled to Paris for the surgery known as trepanning, though her friend Henry More dissuaded her from going through with it.[34] This quite impressive list of attempted cures underscores the severity of Conway's suffering and demonstrates the lengths to which she was prepared to go to alleviate it. Conway's position is a theological "both/and": she accepts suffering, without foreclosing on the possibility of seeking to end it, even to employ the latest known technologies in the attempt.

TECHNOLOGICAL ENHANCEMENT OF THE CREATURE?

Conway's ontology not only makes space for the possibility of transformation of the creature; it makes this the categorical definition of what it means to be Creature; as such, we have an example of a theologically grounded understanding of the nature of human being that can accommodate visions of change, even radical change, that might include bioenhancement technologies. This opens up a unique possible response, theologically and ontologically, to questions of enhancement.

Michael Burdett and Victoria Lorrimar argue that theological responses to the question of human enhancement have gravitated to one or the other of the two poles of "creatureliness" or "deification."[35] Responses centered on creatureliness, often because they take for granted a static view of essences or natures, tend to dismiss the possibility of, or simply morally condemn, the kinds of interventions on the human body that bioenhancement might entail. Responses centered on deification tend to accept at least the theoretical possibility and moral permissibility of enhancement.

In contrast, Conway's concept of creatureliness, as definitively mutable, affirms the possibility of change in the creature. It is, further, morally incumbent on all creatures to transform and, in so doing, more perfectly embody the goodness intended for them by the Creator. As Hutton notes, "The mutability of creatures is, after all, essential to the perfectibility of the created world, for without it creatures could not increase in perfection."[36] Change is the necessary mechanism by which the justice of God is enacted in the world, making possible the restoration of the creature not simply to its original goodness but, as Conway says, "unto a better State than that was in which they were created," for the Good may be pursued ad infinitum.[37]

Yet, these transformations take place without endangering or altering the relationship of Creature to Creator, which remains, as always, defined by the difference between the mutable and immutable. No matter how many steps a creature might ascend on Conway's Ladder, Creature will never become Creator. In such a system, categorical objections to bioenhancement based upon notions of "playing God" simply make no sense. Theologically, then, Conway defies the polarized framework of contemporary theological responses to enhancement; her notion of creatureliness includes mutability, and her notion of transformation precludes deification.

This open-ended sense of permissibility does not cast any direct light on the practical question of what sorts of transformations through the mechanism of bioenhancement might be good or useful or morally permissible; however, Conway's ontology offers us broad hints regarding the way forward in its consideration of what it means to be Creature.

First, her system provides a concept of spiritual-material existence that interprets physical experience as simultaneously spiritual, explicitly resisting the idea that materiality ought to be conceived in terms of endlessly exploitable, manipulable "dead matter." This may serve as a reminder to Christian theologians, engaging in discussion of possible manipulations of our materiality, that what we do with the stuff of which we are made has spiritual implications. This, I suggest, is a stronger *theological* argument for caution than the sort of pragmatic arguments for caution grounded in an appeal to "unintended consequences" of existential threat. Further, Conway's notion of perfectibility includes an explicitly moral dimension, for creatures are meant to aspire toward the Good.

Second, this "vitalism" provides the foundation for an articulation of ontological kinship across what are normally considered ontological boundaries between species. Conway writes that by virtue of sharing one essence, "there remains yet something of Universal Love in all Creatures, one towards another, setting aside that great confusion which hath fallen out since, by reason of Transgression; which certainly must proceed from the same Foundation, viz. in regard of their First Substance and Essence, they were all one and the same Thing, and as it were Parts and Members of one Body."[38] Conway's vision of ontological kinship of creatures can function as a reminder that the human does not exist apart from the rest of creation; considerations of bioenhancement of the human must take this into account.

Finally, her attention to the reality of physical suffering, while potentially problematic in some respects, yields two insights—one we might call a consideration of the particular vulnerabilities of the individual, and the other a consideration of the universal vulnerability of all creatures.

In Conway's ontology, the individual creature never disappears from consideration, even as she explores the essential unity of the ontological category and the kinship it implies. This theology centers the agency of the particular sufferer in both enduring suffering and seeking an end to it. Whether enduring suffering or seeking to alleviate suffering, the common thread for Conway is that the agency of the suffering creature is central, and how the creature responds—whether to turn toward or away from its fundamental orientation toward, and participation in, the Good—is the point. This suggests, for us, that attention to the particularities of the individual, the specific material-spiritual needs of that person, must be central to our theological and ethical consideration of the application of biotechnologies.

At the same time, while we may not want to valorize suffering itself as a spiritual necessity in the way that Conway does, her acceptance that material-spiritual existence contains the ineradicable possibility of suffering is a recognition of a universally shared creaturely vulnerability. In applying Conway's ontology to the question of bioenhancement, we move out of the territory of therapeutic or restorative applications of biotechnology and, therefore, also out of the context of active physical suffering and into what we might call simply universal biological vulnerability.[39] As suggested at the outset, this forms the implicit context of discussions of bioenhancement, for the meaning of such interventions depends upon the implicitly understood context of the limitations and vulnerabilities of present embodiments.

In conclusion, Conway's ontology of Creature provides us with the theological grounding for a nuanced perspective on bioenhancement: open to the possibility of creaturely transformation, oriented to the Good, appreciative of the universal vulnerabilities of all creatures, and aware of the spiritual implications of material transformation. Such a perspective allows for more than a reactionary "no" and better than a reckless "yes." As Anne Conway's own life and thought testifies, we must work out how our creaturely vulnerabilities, and the possibility of suffering implied, offer us opportunity to pursue the Good—through both endurance and transformation.

Notes

1   Sarah Hutton, *Anne Conway: A Woman Philosopher* (Cambridge: Cambridge University Press, 2004), 5; Anne Finch, Viscountess of Conway [aka Anne Conway], *The Principles of the Most Ancient and Modern Philosophy* (London, 1692), https://digital.library.upenn.edu/women/conway/principles/principles.html.

2   Hutton, *Anne Conway*, 2, 3–5.

3   Francis Mercury van Helmont, "To the Reader," in Conway, *Principles*.

4   Quoted in Hutton, *Anne Conway*, 5.

5   Hutton, *Anne Conway*, 7.

6   Hutton, *Anne Conway*, 181: "It was after her encounter with the Quakers that Anne Conway formulated her own explanation of suffering as spiritually medicinal. In so doing she was able to reconcile God's loving goodness with the miseries endured by created beings."

7   The full title and subtitle: *The Principles of the most Ancient and Modern Philosophy concerning God, Christ and the Creatures, viz. of Spirit and Matter in general, whereby may be resolved all those Problems or Difficulties, which neither by the School nor Common Modern Philosophy, nor by the Cartesian, Hobbesian, or Spinosian, could be discussed.*

8   Chapter I, §1. (Here and below, citations to chapters refer to Conway, *Principles*.)

9   Chapter I, §4.

10   Chapters IV and V.

11   Chapter VI, §4 (emphasis original). *Species*, for Conway, is most often her word for "ontological category," not a reference to biological species, though here and elsewhere she employs both senses of the term.

12   Chapter V, §3.

13   Jane Duran, "Conway and Leibniz: The Ideal and the Real," in *An Unconventional History of Western Philosophy: Conversations between Men and Women Philosophers*, ed. Karen Warren (New York: Rowman & Littlefield, 2009), 278.

14   Duran, "Conway and Leibniz," in Warren, *Unconventional History*, 279.

15   Chapter IX, §1.

16   Chapter IX, §2.

17   Elisabeth of Bohemia, in Warren, *Unconventional History*, 162.

18   Chapter VIII, §1.

19   Duran, "Conway and Leibniz," in Warren, *Unconventional History*, 279.

20   Chapter VI, §2.

21   Chapter VI, §3.

22   Chapter VI, §3.

23   Chapter VI, §4.

24   Chapter VI, §5.

25   Chapter VI, §6.

26   Chapter VI, §6.

27   Chapter VII, §1: "Every degree of Sin or Evil hath its Punishment, Grief, and Chastisement annexed to it, in the very Nature of the Thing, by which the Evil is again changed into Good."

28   Chapter VIII, §1.

29   Chapter VII, §1.

30   For further reading on this, see E. S. Kempson, "Anne Conway's Exemplary Engagement with Origenist Thought," *Modern Theology* 38, no. 2 (2022): 389–418; for an argument classifying Hick's theodicy as Origenist rather than Irenaean, see Mark S. M. Scott, "Suffering and Soul-Making: Rethinking John Hick's Theodicy," *Journal of Religion* 90, no. 3 (2010): 313–34.

31   Hutton, *Anne Conway*, 116.

32   Thomas Willis, *De anima brutorum* (London, 1672); quoted in Hutton, *Anne Conway*, 119–20.

33   Hutton, *Anne Conway*, 116. Laura Alexander comments similarly in her analysis in "Anne Conway's Vitalism: A Physico-theological Philosophy," *ANQ: A Quarterly Journal of Short Articles, Notes and Reviews* 32, no. 2 (2019): 93–96.

34   Hutton, *Anne Conway*, 121–22.

35   Michael Burdett and Victoria Lorrimar, "Creatures Bound for Glory: Biotechnological Enhancement and Visions of Human Flourishing," *Studies in Christian Ethics* 32, no. 2 (2019): 241–53.

36   Hutton, *Anne Conway*, 222.

37   Chapter VII, §1.

38   Chapter VII, §3.

39   For a consideration of vulnerability in moral theory and bioethics, see Catriona Mackenzie, Wendy Rogers, and Susan Dodds, eds., *Vulnerability: New Essays in Ethics and Feminist Philosophy* (New York: Oxford University Press, 2014).

3

THE TREE OF LIFE

Aquinas, Disability, and Transhumanism

Miguel J. Romero and Jason T. Eberl

The connection between disability and transhumanism may not be obvious at first blush. While there is a practical consensus on the family of descriptions and proposals that are typically classified under the heading "transhumanism,"[1] the term "disability" is a contested category among contemporary philosophers.[2] In this essay, we adopt an understanding of disability broadly based upon Elizabeth Barnes' "value–neutral model," but adjusted beyond the immanent frame of naturalism to cohere with the realist account of corporal goods provided in Thomistic metaphysics.[3] Understood in this way and for the purpose of comparison, the "disability perspective" will demarcate a rule–based family of descriptions and proposals arising from the justice–promoting solidarity shared among people with physically nonstandard bodies.[4]

The goal of this essay is twofold. The first is to describe one point where the disability perspective and transhumanism intersect: namely, as competing contemporary proposals concerning the significance of our ordinary vulnerability to impairment, illness, and injury.[5] The second is to advance the thesis that our thinking about disability and transhumanism is enriched when considered through the lens of Christian theological anthropology—specifically, through reflection on the Christian account of the vulnerable human body and its condition amid the unfolding drama of the history of grace: original innocence, the present state of corruption, and hope in the bodily resurrection of the dead.

Taking Thomas Aquinas as our primary interlocutor, we contend that the Christian account of the Tree of Life provides a way to harmonize the intuition to affirm the goodness of the human body as given (disability perspective) and the optimistic concern for what the human body could be (transhumanism). Although the Tree of Life offers a principal point of connection between the disability perspective and transhumanism, the Christian story surrounding the Tree of Life is our primary interest. The Tree of Life and the cosmic outlook that anchors its significance are, of course, theological notions derived from the Judeo–Christian scriptures, which Christians take to be an authoritative source of revealed truth, conveyed in a plurality of senses (literal, analogical, anagogical, moral, etc.).[6] Beyond that specifically Christian doctrinal significance, the Tree of Life and the Christian history of grace can function as a kind of thought experiment for those who are not Christians, providing a "just so" story that offers an integrated picture of physical and cognitive differences set in an altogether different and illuminating frame.

APPROACHING DISABILITY AND TRANSHUMANISM VIA CHRISTIANITY

In the first decades of the third millennium, there has been a dramatic increase in the number of philosophers, theologians, and bioethicists taking a scholarly interest in the topics of disability and transhumanism. Typically, the two topics are treated in isolation from each other, where the principles of any specific engagement make it difficult, if not impossible, to engage the topics as part of a larger whole.[7] On the one hand, scholars who aim to advance a broadly transhumanist program tend to dismiss the concerns of disability scholars and advocates as, at best, sentimental and esoteric and, at worst, irrational and regressively idiosyncratic. On the other hand, scholars who aim to advance a broadly anti–ableistic program tend to dismiss the concerns of transhumanist scholars and advocates as, at best, delusional and utopian and, at worst, the dark eugenic harbinger of a rising technofascist global society.

Acknowledging that a certain antagonism exists between these two camps, we claim that a deep connection becomes apparent when scholarly engagement with the topics of transhumanism and disability are framed as extensions of the meliorist/anti-meliorist debate of the past quarter-century.[8] When these camps are framed in that way, as discussed below, two competing accounts become apparent concerning the nature, significance, and implications of the vulnerabilities, limitations, and dependencies of the human body: *eugenic transhumanism* (ETH) and *progenic citra-humanism* (PCH).[9]

Pursuing truth at the intersection of faith and reason, this essay offers a comparative analysis of the basic intuitions, key presumptions, and critical shortcomings of these two camps. It then aims to show how Christianity affirms the central intuitions of each, corrects their respective shortcomings, and enriches each in light of the other. We take Aquinas as our touchstone for the present comparative analysis as he represents this combinatorial approach par excellence: understanding-seeking-faith and faith-seeking-understanding.[10] Aquinas' account of the human being, the human end, and the graced journey of the human being to beatitude provides an illuminative framework for this study.[11] Specifically, reasoning beyond the immanent frame of naturalism, Aquinas' metaphysically realist account of corporal goods (and the privation of those goods) offers an alternative to thin depictions of disability as a good, bad, or mere difference.[12] From the Christian perspective, "good" things can be pursued in a bad way, superficially "bad" things are often revealed to be profound goods, and set within the context of the Christian story—ultimately—there is nothing "mere" or "value-neutral" about the bodily differences that constitute the individual and collective beauty of humanity.

COMPETING ACCOUNTS OF HUMAN NATURE AND FLOURISHING

Though there are other ways of thinking about the characteristics of our corporality, ETH and PCH stand out in the twentieth and twenty-first centuries as rival paradigms at odds for most of the existence of bioethics as a field of discourse.[13] These rival paradigms can be understood as extensions of a conception of human flourishing or "happiness" that dominates late-modern Western consumer capitalist culture:

> *Happiness, thus understood, is a state of only positive feelings. It is therefore a state of freedom from unsatisfied desires and precludes grave apprehensions and fears.* It comes in degrees, as does unhappiness, and everyone on this view wants to be happy in as many aspects of their life as possible. Different individuals in avowing or ascribing happiness may give more or less importance to this or that aspect. But they agree, and on this individual agents in their everyday lives and social scientific researchers are at one, in judging happiness so understood to be a very great good, perhaps the good.[14]

In contemporary Western societies, happiness is understood as a life of unimpeded preference satisfaction, where the individual consumer is free to attain physical and psychological well-being through the satiation of desires and the unfettered power to exclude anything contrary to one's own will. The central privilege mediating this vision of happiness is personal choice, subjective sovereignty. Understood in this way, happiness means maximal freedom from the interests and desires of others and maximal freedom to satiate one's own interests and desires.

The ETH and PCH paradigms come into conflict around the societal implications of their respective preferences. ETH proponents envision and work toward a future where individual preferences will not be constrained or threatened by disabling progenic conditions, one's own or that of another. PCH proponents envision and work toward a present where individual preferences are not constrained or threatened by the eugenic societal consequences of transhumanist aims. Let us explore these paradigms in more detail.

Comparative Analysis of ETH and PCH

Eugenic Transhumanism

ETH fundamentally affirms human bodily potential and expresses a concern to progress, and perhaps even to depart, from the body's present form in favor of a body we can have in the future. It is a cultural extension of the concept of human health and well-being informed by the late nineteenth- and early twentieth-century eugenics movement, arising from the nineteenth-century application of biological *techne* to the practices of medicine.[15] The animating concerns are evolutionary and developmental: human beings considered in light of their temporal context, relations, and interactions. ETH's overarching imperative is to maximize one's own capacity to exercise subjective sovereignty over one's body. Attaining this telos involves affirming the dynamic plasticity of bodily characteristics, which can and should be augmented according to the interests of the sovereign self: morphological freedom is the ultimate form of human flourishing.[16]

ETH's ideological outlook animates, among other things, practices of extreme bodily modification, pharmacological enhancements, utopian technocratic visions, and cultural consumer fetishes characteristic of internet pornography, virtual identities, and social media. It betrays a form of body-self dualism and expressive individualism in which a human being is envisioned as essentially an intellect that occupies a body, which has thrived precisely because of our species' natural aptitude for overcoming the bodily vulnerabilities, limitations, and dependencies of our species through technology, industry, and independence.[17] This view of human anthropology and teleology evinces a low regard for the rights of those who have rare genetic anomalies, abnormal bodily function, or atypical development.

Progenic Citra-humanism

PCH affirms human bodily nature as presently given, expressing a concern to embrace the body we have now. It is a cultural extension of the concept of human health and well-being informed by the late nineteenth- and early twentieth-century ecological movement, arising from mid-to-late nineteenth-century resistance to the centralized, capitalist application of industrial *techne* to common human goods (land, water, air, food production) in a manner that threatened the interests and preference satisfaction of the sovereign individual.[18] The animating concerns are eco-systemic and naturalistically holistic: the human being in general and the human body in particular considered in light of one's environment, sociopolitical context, relations, and interactions. PCH's overarching imperative is to avoid the subjugation and objectification of one's body to the sovereignty of others. Attaining this telos involves affirming the static givenness of bodily characteristics, which should be accommodated according to the interests of the sovereign self.[19]

PCH's polyvalent ideological outlook is unified by its origin in Michel Foucault's critical conceptions of biopower and biopolitics,[20] exemplified in arguments concerning the larger social effects of a too enthusiastic embrace of biomedical enhancement technologies.[21] The human being is envisioned in a reductive sociobiological fashion as a super-primate that happens to have intellect, which has thrived precisely because of our species' natural aptitude for overcoming bodily vulnerabilities, limitations, and dependencies through social cooperation.[22] This view of human anthropology and teleology evinces a high regard for the rights of those who have rare genetic anomalies, abnormal bodily function, or atypical development.

ETH and PCH's Respective Anthropologies

ETH and PCH are respectively founded upon two contradictory anthropological self-understandings, between which the late modern subject vacillates:[23] the former upon a neo-gnostic *angelism* and the latter upon a naturalistic *animalism*. The first, despite disavowing any ontologically immaterial aspect of human nature (i.e., no soul in either the Platonic or the Thomistic senses), views a human being as an essentially disembodied will struggling to subject everything exterior to itself, including the body, to its sovereign dictates. The second, although it may espouse an elevated (even transcendental) notion of health and wellness, views a human being as nothing more than a body that has evolved the illusions of mind and consciousness through the intricate interplay between random genetic mutation and specific ecological niche preferment. Each view, in its own way, captures something true about human nature—yet, even as they do so, each selectively ignores other aspects of human nature.

ETH's angelistic anthropology allows its adherents to envision a future in which a human being may be able to have their cerebrum removed from their dying body and transplanted into a younger and healthier body,[24] transform their organic body into a more advanced cyborg form,[25] or shed their body altogether by having their consciousness uploaded into a cybernetic network[26]—a goal known as "substrate–independence."[27] By contrast, the reductive animalist anthropology that leads the PCH outlook to question both the possibility and the desirability of cyborg transcendence or cybernetic transmutation of mind[28] likewise makes it difficult to imagine an immaterial principle of personhood and individuating identity that coheres, for example, with the ordinary presumptions that predicate discourse about justice and the common good.

Critique of ETH's and PCH's Respective Anthropologies

ETH's angelist characterization of human nature risks stripping us of essential features of our humanity. First and foremost is our *vulnerability* and *finitude,*[29] negligence of which can lead to failure to cultivate "virtues of acknowledged dependence" that are arguably essential for human beings to flourish.[30] Not only to survive vulnerable periods of our lives, but also to mature morally as practical reasoners, we are unavoidably dependent upon others. In turn, others' vulnerability demands that we acknowledge our moral responsibility to promote their flourishing.[31] In short, no individual person is an island unto oneself with respect to one's physical or moral development, and promoting forms of physical enhancement in an attempt to eliminate *any* vulnerability or dependency could have a negative impact on our sense of interpersonal responsibility for each other's well–being. Additionally, while we ought not to seek pain or suffering for its own sake, there is a potential instrumental value to such otherwise negative experiences that may be occluded by seeking to eliminate various vulnerabilities.[32]

By contrast, PCH's animalist account affirms our essential embodiment with all of the characteristics just described.[33] Yet, animalism's reductive construal of human nature fails to do justice to the full dimensionality of human personhood, precisely because animalism separates human personhood from human animality in arguing that the latter is what we fundamentally are, with the former as a mere "phase" of our existence.[34] Critics of animalism contend that one's existence and survival as a *person* is "what matters to us";[35] thus, any account of human nature that "directly connects what is most important to us and about us with what we most fundamentally are"[36] is all the better for doing so. As we will show, Thomistic anthropology—in which human beings are understood as a hylomorphic unity of intellect and matter composing a "rational animal" endowed with (among other essential qualities) volitional freedom—offers a *via media* that provides a more complete account of human beings as persons who are neither angels (i.e., disembodied intellects and wills) nor merely animals.[37]

CHRISTIAN THEO-PHILOSOPHICAL CRITIQUE OF ETH AND PCH

Amid the debate between eugenic transhumanists—such as Nick Bostrom, Allen Buchanan, and Max Moore[38]—and progenic citra-humanists—such as Francis Fukuyama, Michael Sandel, and Leon Kass[39]—Catholic theologians and philosophers have a speculative resource in the tradition of Christian reflection on references to the Tree of Life in Scripture.[40] The biblical depiction of the Tree of Life places it along a line that traces the entire sweep of revealed human history: original justice; original sin; the fall with its concomitant spiritual and corporal wounds; the incarnation, passion, and resurrection of Jesus Christ; sacramental grace; and Christian hope in bodily resurrection and final beatitude. The primary lessons from the biblical accounts of the Tree of Life that pertain to the current discussion are the following:

- Human beings are presented as naturally mortal, vulnerable, and dependent creatures.
- There is an affirmation of the inherent goodness of our natural mortality, vulnerability, and dependency, which are integral to the prelapsarian perfection of the human being.
- In the state of original innocence, there was a natural means provided to attain preternatural bodily well-being.
- The desire for preternatural corporal perfection is not evil, but it can be disordered and harmful when separated from friendship with God.

As we will discuss in more detail via Aquinas below, within the Christian story we see an affirmation of the core intuition of PCH (the goodness of the human body as given) and the core intuition of ETH (the goodness of the human body as it could be). However,

Christianity parts ways with both on two points: their respective conceptions of human nature and the human good. Against the reductive animalism of PCH and the gnostic angelism of ETH stands the Christian understanding of our composite nature: an incorruptible intellectual soul existing in and through a corruptible body as the substantial form of that body.[41] Further, for both PCH and ETH, the good of human beings in relation to their bodies is an immanent, this-worldly goal or aim. For PCH the goal is a progenic sociopolitical order where constraint of *what-we-are* is taken to be the constraint of persons; while for ETH the goal is a eugenic biotechnic order where constraint of *what-we-could-be* is taken to be constraint of the species.

As Christians see it, our given nature predicates the greatest good and final perfection of human beings in relation to our Creator. The journey from *what-we-are* to *what-we-could-be* is a change capacitated and facilitated by an unmerited, supernatural gift called grace, a cooperative, noncompetitive endowment: *grace does not destroy nature; it perfects it*. It involves a change that affirms and reconciles the core intuitions of both PCH and ETH while preserving a distinctive anthropological, teleological, and soteriological vision.

Aquinas, Transhumanism, and the Disability Perspective

According to Aquinas, the human being is an incarnate intellectual creature, capable of knowing and loving God. Unambiguously rooted in the principles of Christian revelation, Thomistic theological anthropology recognizes that the human being has a twofold end, natural and supernatural: moral virtue in this life and the beatific vision of divine glory in the life to come. The perfection of human beings by divine grace, on this view, cannot be separated from the fact of our corporality, with its inherent vulnerability and mortality, and concomitant dependence on each other and the goods of the earth. This was as true of human beings in the preternatural condition of original grace as it is of us today, wounded by sin and living amid the consequences of the fall.

At the beginning of the twenty-first century, the anthropological outlook and moral ends of transhumanism's (ETH-framed) technological imperative present an alternative vision of human flourishing, one of perpetual technological progress with no defined omega (understood by way of the immanent frame of naturalism). It is an outlook that eschews the value of humanity's embodied condition in calling for an ultimate virtual transcendence of our bodies. Christians, by contrast, believe that a human life is only intelligible in light of the grace-capacitated ultimate end of the human being, the beatific vision of God and final resurrection of the dead. Even as Christians affirm the intuition that pain (in body or in spirit) is often—though not always—associated with the impairments, ills, and injuries of this life and that, further, to be free of such pains is a worthy hope, it is a fundamental Christian truth that the privation of corporal goods does not undermine the goodness of corporeality and that the final resurrection will be a resurrection of the human body that is proper and particular to each individual person. For that reason, amid the course of this earthly life, Christians live in hope of a divinely wrought spiritual-cum-corporal healing and eschatological transformation, in which the limits of corporality are perfected without denying our essentially embodied nature. Aquinas' understanding of our innate creaturely vulnerabilities in relation to human beings' twofold end provides a way for Christians, from a theologically informed disability perspective, to critically engage some of the metaphysical claims and presumptions of transhumanism.

The anthropological outlook and moral ends of the (PCH-framed) disability perspective likewise present an alternative vision of human flourishing. The justice-based concerns that drive the disability perspective are indeed urgent in the contemporary sociopolitical context where persons who have an impairment or disability continue to be ignored, alienated, socially excluded, and systematically erased from the human family through selective screening. Nevertheless, even as Christians (physically impaired and unimpaired, able-bodied and those who have a disability) rightly find common cause with the justice-promoting solidarity shared among people with physically nonstandard bodies, it is a fundamental Christian truth that the wound of sin has set the body of every human being in a state of profound disorder and, further, that the manifold goods that come from our ongoing work for a just sociopolitical order will, ultimately, fall short of the perfect good, everlasting communion, and consummate happiness of final beatitude. Moreover, for Christians, the various kinds and degrees of impairment to which every human being is vulnerable are understood to have a significance that stretches beyond this life. Aquinas' understanding of the corporeal consequences of original sin and the eschatological significance of our corporal wounds (in light of the glorified wounds of Christ) provide a way for Christians, from a theologically informed assessment of transhumanist intuitions, to challenge the immanent frame of naturalism that is standard to the contemporary disability perspective.

Aquinas on the Human Body in the State of Original Innocence

In QQ. 94–102 of the Prima Pars of his *Summa theologiae*, Aquinas outlines the providentially ordained proper function of human beings in the state of innocence: the condition of the human soul, the human body, and the primeval paradisal abode.[42] He distinguishes between the integrity of human nature in the state of innocence and the corruption of human nature in the state of sin.[43] For Aquinas, in this context, the distinction between integrity and corruption pertains to the operation of a thing, not its nature.[44] This distinction is important because it underscores why Aquinas' understanding of impairment, illness, and injury is formally and categorically irreconcilable (and even critically at odds) with the eugenic biomedical presumptions and chauvinistic norms that construe bodily difference as "deviance from species," bodily damage as "perversion of nature," and a spectrum of bodily defects as sufficient cause for formal disqualification from the due regard of justice.[45]

In the state of innocence, the human soul was properly disposed to perfectly command and use the human body, so that the faculties and passions of the body were not a hindrance to the soul.[46] Aquinas is keen to clarify, however, that this subjection of the body to the soul and of the lower powers to reason was not due to something proper to human nature; otherwise it would have remained after sin. Rather, the preternatural functioning of the body was among the benefits of original grace.[47]

Aquinas' account of the human body in the state of innocence is extended when he considers the dominion attributed to humanity in Genesis 1:26. For Aquinas, the truth–grounded and truth–oriented goodness of humanity overflowed into a harmonious manner of relating with fellow creatures.[48] It is in this context that Aquinas considers if there would have been equality between human beings in the state of innocence—specifically, "equality" in the sense of uniformity, the absence of diversity and individuating differences.[49] Aquinas answers no, there would not have been equality between human beings; rather, Aquinas contends that there must have been an expansive inequality and diversity among members of the human species. It is important to keep in mind what Aquinas is presuming as he navigates this question—namely, his view that the perfection of the universe consists in the diversity of creatures[50] and his conviction that every human being is formed in the image and toward the likeness of the triune God.[51] On that basis, given the ordinary entailments of biological procreation, from the outset Aquinas takes for granted that there were differences of sex (between reproductive partners) and age (between parents and children).

Reasoning further, he argues that there likely would have been a diversity of bodies insofar as primitive humanity in the state of innocence would not have been exempt from the ordinary operations and effects of the natural world. For Aquinas, differences in food, climate, and even the subtle influence of cosmic forces (e.g., the movements of the stars) would have caused individuating differences. He notes, for example, that there would have been manifold differences of bodily vigor or strength (*robustiores*), size (*maiores*), physical beauty (*pulchriores*), and overall bodily configuration (*complexionati*; i.e., relevant to physiological temperament, personal disposition, and outward appearance).[52]

In laying out this kaleidoscopic vision of humanity in the state of innocence—variegate in every conceivable way—Aquinas is clear that there would have been no defect of body or fault of sin in those who happened to be physically weak, small in stature, superficially less comely, or who simply did not seem to "fit in" at first blush (due to an unusual temperament, appearance, or disposition). According to Aquinas, a diversity of bodies would have been integral to the beauty of primitive humanity in the state of innocence.[53] In essence, inequality between persons would have been the providential exaltation of each person's individual dignity and would be predicate to that person's graced destiny as a being formed in the image and toward the likeness of the triune God: so that "the beauty of order would the more shine forth among humanity."[54]

Preservation of Humanity and the Tree of Life

With this background, Aquinas next discusses the preservation and protection of the human body in the state of innocence. His concern throughout is to make sense of the Christian doctrine that humanity on the whole became subject to suffering, bodily impairment, and death as consequence of original sin. The challenge is to show the integral coherence of the Christian affirmation of the goodness of the human body *as given* (i.e., even as we know it now in the state of corruption: mortal, passible, vulnerable, and dependent) in relation to what Christians affirm about the body *as it was and will be* (in the graced state of original innocence and the glorified state of the resurrection). He does this through a set of distinctions (concerning *immortality* and *impassibility*), a discussion of what is needed to sustain the animal life of the human body, and then a discussion of what was given in the state of innocence to sustain the life of the human body.

Aquinas begins by mapping the notion of immortality, drawing upon a metaphysical frame established previously concerning the composite nature of the human being.[55] On the understanding that the mortality of animal life consists in its susceptibility to material corruption, wherein the formal cause of a thing is separated from its material cause, Aquinas stipulates that immortality implies incorruptibility. Understood in that way, there are three ways a thing can be incorruptible:[56] first, by nature, as with creatures that have no material form (i.e., angels) and simple material creatures that are in potentiality to only one form (i.e., heavenly bodies); second, when the incorruptible form of a naturally corruptible composite thing is inherently disposed to preserve itself from corruption (i.e., the intellectual soul, partaking in the beatific vision and the glory of the resurrection); and, third, when a composite creature like the human being remains near or intimate with the ongoing creative act of its Creator (our efficient cause). So conceived, Aquinas explains that the third case applies to the human being in the state of innocence—whereby the formal power of the intellectual soul to animate and preserve its body was supernaturally enhanced by its ongoing, intimate submission to the divine source of its own creaturely existence.

Having established the sense in which an animal body can be immortal (i.e., incorruptible), Aquinas draws upon previous arguments[57] and reiterates the sense in which "impassibility" can be attributed to a naturally corruptible creature being supernaturally sustained in a state of bodily incorruption.[58] He distinguishes between two ways in which things are said to be "passible."[59] The first is when a thing is subject to (i.e., it can "suffer") a change to its natural disposition by some external effect. In this sense, humanity was impassible in the state of innocence. The other concerns change more generally, including the process in which the nature of a thing is perfected individually and collectively over time. Understood in that way, primitive humanity was not subject to external effects that could definitively undermine the natural balanced disposition of the body, while remaining sensitive to external effects and capable of perfective change (i.e., both individual growth and the biological evolution of the species).[60]

For Aquinas, the best way to understand the natural disposition of the human body is to consider the intellectual soul, which is its form.[61] To wit, the intellectual soul is not naturally gifted with knowledge of truth (as are angels). Rather, human beings learn by way of sensation. For this reason, it is necessary that the intellectual soul be united with a body capable of sensation. Aquinas understands sensation to be the perception of contraries, which means that the most fitting body for the human being is one that is sensitive and thus vulnerable to material corruption.[62]

We can triangulate some further entailments of Aquinas' view. First, because sensation is a matter of degree and physical pain is the excess of sensation, primitive humanity would have experienced physical pain in certain circumstances—although it would not have been attended by the spiritual sorrow typically associated with "suffering." Second, the human body in the state of innocence would have been vulnerable to everyday ordinary injuries and ills (cuts, broken bones, sunburns, infections, etc.)—none of those things, of course, could undermine the natural disposition of the human body in its operation as the sensing organ of the intellectual soul.

In tracing Aquinas' view, it is important to notice how the soft and sensitive body of the human being was preserved from extraordinary injuries of the sort that could definitively undermine the body's balanced disposition and operation. Aquinas speculates that the preternatural rational faculties of humanity would have protected against foreseeable threats and that divine providence could have protected against what was unforeseeable.[63] In principle, then, the presence of occasional bodily impairments, illnesses, and injuries cannot be excluded from the state of original innocence. Aquinas affirms this in his discussion of the human being's tendency toward corruptive dissolution, which the Tree of Life was given to mitigate:

> The intellectual soul requires a body [that is] corruptible by force of its matter. . . . God, however, provided in this case by applying a remedy against death.

Aquinas then asks what was needed to preserve the human being's corruptible animal life in the state of innocence. He answers quickly, on the authority of Scripture: food.[64] Beyond ordinary food, which energizes ordinary human activity and growth, a different kind of food was needed to preserve and strengthen the human body against its natural tendency toward material corruption.[65] For the ordinary sustenance of life was given the trees of paradise, and for the preservation and strengthening of life was given the Tree of Life:

> In old age, [ordinary food] does not suffice even for [growth and preservation]; whereupon the body declines, and finally dies from natural causes. Against this defect man was provided with a remedy in the tree of life; for its effect was to strengthen the force of the species against the weakness resulting from the admixture of extraneous nutriment. Wherefore Augustine says . . . *The tree of life, like a drug, warded off all bodily corruption.*[66]

Although the Tree of Life provided whatever was needed to prevent death, it was not on its own the cause of immortality. For Aquinas, the animating principle of the integrity, growth, and preservation of the human body is the intellectual soul. The Tree of Life provided the human body with the matter that the intellectual soul needed in order to conserve the body. Because the Tree of Life and the nourishment it provided were finite, the benefits were likewise finite.[67]

With Aquinas' view in hand, it is important to distinguish between the corporal integrity preserved by the Tree of Life and the late-modern anthropological "norm" toward which we are tempted in the wake of biomedicine's eugenic caricature of what it means to have a "perfect" or "good" human body. Specifically, by Aquinas' reckoning, in preserving the human body from material dissolution and fortifying the body against age-related corruption, the Tree of Life would not have undermined or counteracted the global diversity of human bodies in the state of innocence.

In other words, the individuating effects of the natural world on the human body—via food, climate, and subtle cosmic forces—would have been strengthened by the integrating power of the intellectual soul in the state of grace, and those differences would not have been erased by the remedial and anti-corruptive nourishment provided by the Tree of Life. Primitive humanity thus would have manifested a breathtaking diversity of bodies—intimate with the divine source of its own existence and free from any corporal defect that could undermine the operation of the body as the soul's organ of sensation. Some individuals would have been physically strong, others comparatively weak; some would be large in stature, others small in stature; some would have been physically beautiful, others less so; and throughout there would have been a magnificent variety in outward appearances, personalities, and temperamental dispositions.

Conclusion—Eschatological Considerations

As noted above, a form of gnostic angelism primarily characterizes the ETH view of humanity's evolutionary omega—namely, total morphological freedom involving either an unlimited transmutation of bodily forms or complete independence from corporality altogether. Whereas, the PCH perspective, on a narrow nontheological understanding, considers human embodiment, with its concomitant vulnerability and limitations, to be indelible marks of the human condition. Reflecting upon Aquinas' consideration of the postresurrection human body reveals again a middle-ground position in line with his view of human nature in the prelapsarian state.

Aquinas contends that the human soul (due to its intellective and volitional capacities) is essentially immaterial and thereby incorruptible—that is, capable of persisting in the absence of the body it naturally informs.[68] He considers, however, the soul to be incomplete in this interim state after death, contending that it "longs" for reunion with its body.[69] This reunion is effected by divine fiat at the general resurrection with the result that each human soul will perfectly inform matter supplied to it by God, resulting in what St. Paul refers to as a "glorified body."[70] What St. Paul means by the "glorified body" has been subject to both gnostic and hylomorphic interpretations. With respect to the latter, Aquinas clearly affirms that a human person's resurrected and glorified body will be material, but with abilities—e.g., impassibility, subtlety, agility, and clarity—that surpass our current embodiment.[71]

Disability scholars who accept the Thomistic hylomorphic view of human personhood have discussed the central question of whether physical or cognitive disabilities will persist as constitutive of the postresurrection embodied person.[72] Responses turn on further questions regarding the "perfection" (or "wholeness") of the human person and what is required to experience the beatific vision—that is, loving union with God.

In his *Commentary on the Gospel of John*, Aquinas underscores the significance of the palpable wounds of the resurrected Christ.[73] There and elsewhere,[74] Aquinas teaches that Christ's glorified wounds challenge Christians to a different way of thinking about the wounds we bear in this life. Aquinas is clear that there is no contradiction between the traces of wounds and the perfection of resurrection glory. On that basis, he speculates on the eschatological significance of our wounds, concluding with Augustine that those wounds that were born in a participatory communion with wounds of Christ will remain as traces—not in a manner that would hinder, but as everlasting trophies—and that "a certain kind of beauty will shine in them, in the body, though not of the body."[75]

The upshot of this analysis is that the diversity of human physical and cognitive abilities evidenced in humanity's postlapsarian condition should not be simply categorized as endemic consequences of "the fall" that fundamentally disrupted humanity's relationship not only to the rest of the created world but also to our own embodied nature. Hence, we should not be quick to categorize physical and cognitive disabilities as simply concomitant with humanity's postlapsarian condition, but—as consideration of the Thomistic account of the Tree of Life and the history of grace directs us—to view purported "disabilities" within a wider framework of human anthropology, soteriology, and eschatology to arrive at an account of what physical and cognitive traits comprise humanity's essential nature. Our hypothesis is that such traits will be quite small in number and quite general in description, allowing for a wide range of manifestations of humanity's essential nature and supernatural dignity as rational animal and image of God.

NOTES

1   See Max More, "The Philosophy of Transhumanism," in *The Transhumanist Reader: Classical and Contemporary Essays on the Science, Technology, and Philosophy of the Human Future*, ed. Max More and Natasha Vita-More (Malden, Mass.: Wiley-Blackwell, 2013), 3–17; see also https://www.humanityplus.org.

2   See Kevin Timpe, "Denying a Unified Concept of Disability," *Journal of Medicine and Philosophy* 47, no. 5 (2022): 583–96.

3   See Elizabeth Barnes, *The Minority Body: A Theory of Disability* (Oxford: Oxford University Press, 2016); and n. 12 below.

4   See Barnes, *Minority Body*, 38–53.

5   The fact that these distinct families of descriptions and proposals can be compared formally should not be taken to imply that we consider there to be parity between the two, in either the veracity of description or the ends sought. Rather, as we intend to argue, the divergent anthropological, teleological, and soteriological visions of the disability and transhumanist perspectives have critical shortcomings that can be remedied when brought into conversation with each other by way of the Christian tradition.

6   See Thomas Aquinas, *Summa theologiae* (hereafter "STh") Ia, q. 1, a. 10; trans. English Dominican Fathers (New York: Benziger, 1948).

7   For an astute overview and critical intervention into the point of intersection, see Melinda Hall, *The Bioethics of Enhancement: Transhumanism, Disability, and Biopolitics* (Lanham, Md.: Lexington Books, 2017). See also Miriam Eilers, Katrin Grüber, and Christoph Rehmann-Sutter, eds., *The Human Enhancement Debate and Disability: New Bodies for a Better Life* (New York: Palgrave Macmillan, 2014).

8   See Arthur Caplan, "Good, Better, or Best?" in *Human Enhancement*, ed. Julian Savulescu and Nick Bostrom (Oxford: Oxford University Press, 2009), 199–210.

9   The purpose of these provisional labels is to facilitate comparison between schools of thought that, respectively, defy simplistic classification: "eugenic" refers to "good, better, improved" intrinsic human qualities oriented toward creating a "trans-" (i.e., "on the other side of") humanity's current condition; whereas the term "progenic" refers to "for, toward, in favor of" current intrinsic human qualities oriented toward maintaining a "citra-" (i.e., "on this side of") humanity's current condition.

10   See Leo XIII, *Aeterni patris* (Vatican City: Libreria Editrice Vaticana, 1879); and John Paul II, *Fides et ratio* (Vatican City: Libreria Editrice Vaticana, 1998), nn. 43–45, 64–74.

11   For interpretation and engagement with Aquinas' theology focused on disability, see Miguel J. Romero, "Aquinas on the *corporis infirmitas*: Broken Flesh and the Grammar of Grace," in *Disability in the Christian Tradition: A Reader*, ed. Brian Brock and John Swinton (Grand Rapids: Eerdmans, 2012); "The Happiness of 'Those Who Lack the Use of Reason,'" *Thomist* 80, no. 1 (2016): 49–96; "Intellectual Disability, Spanish Colonialism, and the Disappearance of a Medieval Account of Persons Who Lack the Use of Reason," in *Disability in Medieval Christian Philosophy and Theology*, ed. Scott M. Williams (New York: Routledge, 2020), 134–78.

12   As mentioned above, in this essay we adopt a modified version of Elizabeth Barnes' "value-neutral model." Barnes' value-neutral model of disability holds that, although determined by objective physical features that distinguish individual bodies (38), "disability" is a social distinction constructed from rules for making judgements about group solidarity employed by the disability rights movement (43–46). So conceived, disability is a form of mere-bodily-difference (neither inherently a "bad difference" nor inherently a "good difference"), analogous to sex or race, and essentially neutral with respect to personal well-being: hence, disability "may be good for you, it may be bad for you, it may be utterly indifferent for you—depending on what it is combined with" (98). See Barnes, *Minority Body*. Drawing upon the realist account of corporal goods provided by Aquinas, we have adopted a modified version of the "value-neutral model" that retains the strengths of Barnes' proposal but that can also be extended beyond the immanent frame of naturalism. On our view, physical and cognitive impairments are best understood as privations of capacities that are conducive to human flourishing but that do not inexorably result in disability or undermine the possibility of human flourishing; nor do impairments or disabilities diminish the unique dignity, embodied identity, or experiences of persons with them. For further discussion supporting the understanding of disability we adopt here,

see Nicholas Colgrove, "The (In)compatibility of the Privation Theory of Evil and the Mere-Difference View of Disability," *National Catholic Bioethics Quarterly* 20, no. 2 (2020): 329–48; and Jason T. Eberl, "Disability, Enhancement, and Flourishing," *Journal of Medicine and Philosophy* 47, no. 5 (2022): 597–611.

13   See Miguel J. Romero, "Disability, Catholic Questions, and the Quandaries of Biomedicine and Secular Society," *The National Catholic Bioethics Quarterly* 20, no. 2 (2020): 286. See also Tom Koch, "The Difference that Difference Makes: Bioethics and the Challenge of 'Disability,'" *Journal of Medicine and Philosophy* 29, no. 6 (2004): 697–716; and Susan Wendell, "Toward a Feminist Theory of Disability," *Hypatia* 4, no. 2 (1989): 104–24.

14   Alasdair MacIntyre, *Ethics in the Conflicts of Modernity* (New York: Cambridge University Press, 2016), 196.

15   See Daniel J. Kevles, *In the Name of Eugenics: Genetics and the Uses of Human Heredity* (Cambridge, Mass.: Harvard University Press, 1985); Paul A. Lombardo, *A Century of Eugenics in America: From the Indiana Experiment to the Human Genome Era* (Bloomington: Indiana University Press, 2011); Lennard Davis, *The Disability Studies Reader*, 2nd ed. (New York: Routledge, 2006), viii–xv and 231–42; and Dan Goodley, *Dis/ability Studies: Theorising Disablism and Ableism* (New York: Routledge, 2014).

16   See Anders Sandberg, "Morphological Freedom—Why We Not Just Want It, but Need It," in More and Vita-More, *Transhumanist Reader*.

17   See Patrick Lee and Robert P. George, *Body-Self Dualism in Contemporary Ethics and Politics* (New York: Cambridge University Press, 2009); and O. Carter Snead, *What It Means to Be Human: The Case for the Body in Public Bioethics* (Cambridge, Mass.: Harvard University Press, 2020).

18   See Hans-Martin Sass, "Fritz Jahr's 1927 Concept of Bioethics," *Kennedy Institute of Ethics Journal* 17, no. 4 (2008): 279–95; and Henk ten Have, "Potter's Notion of Bioethics," *Kennedy Institute of Ethics Journal* 22, no. 1 (2012): 59–82. See also Van Rensselaer Potter, "Bioethics: The Science of Survival," *Perspectives in Biology and Medicine* 14, no. 2 (1970): 127–53; and Daniel Callahan, "Bioethics as a Discipline," *Hastings Center Studies* 1, no. 1 (1973): 66–73.

19   See Michael Sandel, *The Case against Perfection: Ethics in the Age of Genetic Engineering* (Cambridge, Mass.: Harvard University Press, 2009).

20   See Michel Foucault, *Madness and Civilization: A History of Insanity in the Age of Reason*, trans. Richard Howard (New York: Vintage Books, 1965); and *The Birth of the Clinic: An Archaeology of Medical Perception* (New York: Vintage Books, 1994).

21 See, for example, Bill McKibben, *Enough: Staying Human in an Engineered Age* (New York: Times Books, 2003); Carl Elliott, *Better than Well: American Medicine Meets the American Dream* (New York: W. W. Norton, 2003); and Francis Fukuyama, *Our Posthuman Future: Consequences of the Biotechnology Revolution* (New York: Picador, 2003).

22 See, for example, Eric T. Olson, *The Human Animal: Personal Identity without Psychology* (New York: Oxford University Press, 1997); Edward O. Wilson, *Sociobiology: The New Synthesis* (Cambridge, Mass.: Harvard University Press, 1975).

23 See Blaise Pascal, *Pensées and Other Writings*, trans. Honor Levi (Oxford: Oxford University Press, 1995), nn. 154 (38), 557 (128). See also Reinhard Hütter, "Body Politics beyond Angelism and Animalism: The Human Passions and Their Irreducible Spiritual Dimension," in *Dust Bound for Heaven: Explorations in the Theology of Thomas Aquinas* (Grand Rapids: Eerdmans, 2012), 75–101; *Bound for Beatitude: A Thomistic Study in Eschatology and Ethics* (Washington, D.C.: Catholic University of America Press, 2019), 153–55.

24 Cerebral transplant is not a novel idea of transhumanists but a thought experiment that philosophers have utilized for several decades; for a recent cerebrum-based view of personal identity, see Jeff McMahan, *The Ethics of Killing: Problems at the Margins of Life* (New York: Oxford University Press, 2002). A perhaps more feasible, but still arguably problematic, proposal involves transplanting one's entire head; see Xiaoping Ren and Sergio Canavero, "HEAVEN in the Making: Between the Rock (the Academe) and a Hard Case (a Head Transplant)," *AJOB Neuroscience* 8, no. 4 (2017): 200–205. For a response to this proposal, see Jason T. Eberl, "Whose Head, Which Body?" *AJOB Neuroscience* 8, no. 4 (2017): 221–23.

25 See Andy Clark, *Natural-Born Cyborgs: Minds, Technologies and the Future of Human Intelligence* (New York: Oxford University Press, 2003).

26 See Ray Kurzweil, *The Singularity Is Near: When Humans Transcend Biology* (New York: Viking, 2005).

27 See Randal A. Koene, "Uploading to Substrate-Independent Minds," in More and Vita-More, *Transhumanist Reader*.

28 See David B. Hershenov, "Why Transhumanists Can't Survive the Death of Their Bodies?" *Ethics, Medicine and Public Health* 10 (2019): 102–10.

29 See Gerald P. McKenny, "Enhancements and the Ethical Significance of Vulnerability," in *Enhancing Human Traits: Ethical and Social Implications*, ed. Erik Parens (Washington, D.C.: Georgetown University Press, 1998), 223, 235. Cf. McKenny, *To Relieve the Human Condition: Bioethics, Technology, and the Body* (Albany: SUNY Press, 1997); Brent Waters, *From Human to Posthuman: Christian Theology and Technology in a*

Postmodern World (Burlington, Vt.: Ashgate, 2006), 60–67, 118–19; Thierry Magnin, "Vulnerability at the Heart of the Ethical Implications of New Biotechnologies," *Human and Social Studies* 4, no. 3 (2015): 13–25.

30   Alasdair MacIntyre, *Dependent Rational Animals: Why Human Beings Need the Virtues* (Chicago: Open Court, 1999).

31   Jason T. Eberl, "Cultivating the Virtue of Acknowledged Responsibility," *Proceedings of the American Catholic Philosophical Association* 82 (2008): 249–61.

32   Jason T. Eberl, "Religious and Secular Perspectives on the Value of Suffering," *National Catholic Bioethics Quarterly* 12, no. 2 (2012): 251–61.

33   Key philosophical articulations and defenses of animalism include Olson, *Human Animal*; and Paul F. Snowdon, *Persons, Animals, Ourselves* (New York: Oxford University Press, 2014). A recent collection of defenses and critiques of animalism can be found in Stephan Blatti and Paul F. Snowdon, eds., *Animalism: New Essays on Persons, Animals, and Identity* (New York: Oxford University Press, 2016). For a critique of animalism from a Thomistic hylomorphic perspective, see Jason T. Eberl, *The Nature of Human Persons: Metaphysics and Bioethics* (Notre Dame: University of Notre Dame Press), ch. 4.

34   Olson, *Human Animal*, 25, 29–30.

35   Derek Parfit, *Reasons and Persons* (New York: Oxford University Press, 1984).

36   Lynne Rudder Baker, *Persons and Bodies: A Constitution View* (New York: Cambridge University Press, 2000), 164.

37   For a fuller articulation and defense of Thomistic hylomorphism, see Eberl, *Nature of Human Persons*.

38   See Nick Bostrom, *Superintelligence: Paths, Dangers, Strategies* (New York: Oxford University Press, 2016); Allen Buchanan, *Beyond Humanity? The Ethics of Biomedical Enhancement* (New York: Oxford University Press, 2013); More, "Philosophy of Transhumanism," in More and Vita-More, *Transhumanist Reader*.

39   See Fukuyama, *Our Posthuman Future*; Sandel, *Case against Perfection*; Leon R. Kass and the President's Council on Bioethics, *Beyond Therapy: Biotechnology and the Pursuit of Happiness* (New York: Harper Perennial, 2003).

40   Gen 2:9, 3:22–24; Prov 3:18, 11:30, 13:12, 15:4; John 3:16–17, 5:13, 6:35, 14:6, 17:3; Rev 2:7, 22:1–19.

41   See STh Ia, q. 76.

42   The interpretive line taken in this essay is compatible with the Thomistic account of the biological evolution of terrestrial life. For an introduction

to the Thomistic account of evolution, which reconciles Christian doctrine on the historicity of an original human being and the doctrine of original sin with contemporary science, see Nicanor Austriaco, James Brent, Thomas Davinport, and John Baptist Ku, eds., *Thomistic Evolution*, 2nd ed. (Providence, R.I.: Cluny Media, 2019).

43   STh Ia, q. 94, a. 2.

44   See STh Ia, q. 93, a. 4, read in light of q. 48, a. 4.

45   See Romero, "Aquinas on the *corporis infirmitas*," in Brock and Swinton, *Disability in the Christian Tradition*, 103–12.

46   STh Ia, q. 95, a. 2.

47   STh Ia, q. 95, a. 1.

48   STh Ia, q. 96, aa. 1–2.

49   STh Ia, q. 96, a. 3.

50   STh Ia, a. 47, aa. 1–2.

51   STh Ia, a. 93, aa. 1, 4, 7, 9.

52   STh Ia, q. 96, a. 3.

53   See Miguel J. Romero, "The Goodness and Beauty of Our Fragile Flesh: Moral Theologians and Our Engagement with Disability," *Journal of Moral Theology* 6, no. 2 (2017): 231–43. For an extended engagement with Aquinas' inchoate aesthetic theory, see Christopher Scott Sevier, *Aquinas on Beauty* (London: Lexington Books, 2015); see also Sevier, "Aquinas on the Relation of Goodness to Beauty," *De Medio Aevo* 2, no. 2 (2013): 103–26.

54   STh Ia, q. 75, a. 4; q. 76, a. 1; q. 96, a. 3 *ad* 3.

55   STh Ia, q. 97, a. 1.

56   STh Ia, q. 97, a. 1.

57   STh Ia, q. 48, a. 4; q. 75, aa. 2, 6; q. 79, aa. 2, 4; q. 95, a. 2.

58   STh Ia, q. 97, a. 2.

59   STh Ia, q. 97, a. 2.

60   STh Ia, q. 22, a. 4; q. 73, a.1, *ad* 3.

61   STh Ia, q. 76, a. 5; *De Malo*, q. 5, a. 5, resp. and *ad* 9.

62   STh Ia, q. 91, a. 3.

63   STh Ia, q. 97, a. 2 *ad* 4.

64   Aquinas notes that the need for food was fitting for the *animal* bodily life of primitive humanity in the state of innocence but that food would not be necessary for *spiritual* bodily life that Christians anticipate after the general resurrection. STh Ia, q. 97, a. 3. For further elucidation of the state of the glorified resurrected body, see Eberl, *Nature of Human Persons*, ch. 7.

65   *De Malo*, q. 5, a. 5, resp. and *ad* 9.

66   STh Ia, q. 97, a. 4 (emphasis added).

67   STh Ia, q. 97, a. 4.

68   STh Ia, qq. 75–76.

69   See Aquinas, *Compendium theologiae* (CTh), bk. I, ch. 151; *Summa contra gentiles* (SCG), bk. IV, ch. 79.

70   Phil 3:20–21; 1 Cor 42–44. See also Aquinas, STh Supp., q. 81, a. 4; SCG, bk. IV, q. 83; CTh, bk. I, ch. 156.

71   See SCG, bk. IV, ch. 84–85; cf. STh Supp., qq. 82–85.

72   See Paul Gondreau, "Disability, the Healing of Infirmity, and the Theological Virtue of Hope: A Thomistic Approach," *Journal of Moral Theology* 6, no. 2 (2017): 70–111; Terrence Ehrman, "Disability and Resurrection Identity," *New Blackfriars* 96, no. 1066 (2015): 723–38; Kevin Timpe, "Disabled Beatitude," in *The Lost Sheep in Philosophy of Religion: New Perspectives on Disability, Gender, Race, and Animals*, ed. Blake Hereth and Kevin Timpe (New York: Routledge, 2020), 241–63; and Bryan R. Cross, "A Thomistic, Non-ableist Conception of Impairment and Disability," *National Catholic Bioethics Quarterly* 20, no. 2 (2020): 233–42. See also Romero, "Aquinas on the *corporis infirmitas*," in Brock and Swinton, *Disability in the Christian Tradition*; and Romero, "Aquinas on Disability, Deification, and Beatitude" (forthcoming).

73   Aquinas, *Commentary on the Gospel of John*, ch. 20, lect. 6, n. 2557.

74   STh IIIa, q. 54, a. 4; q. 55, aa. 5–6.

75   STh IIIa, q. 54, a. 4.

4

ONTOLOGY: WHERE IT COMES IN AND HOW IT MATTERS

A Conversation between Friends

Jonathan Tran and Jeffrey P. Bishop

In the following, moral theologians Jonathan Tran and Jeffrey P. Bishop engage in a conversation about the role ontology plays in ethical disagreements about disability and personhood. The conversation is very much one between friends. That is, here are two people who share deep agreements but differ at significant points. The differences clarify and interestingly complicate the agreements and their implications. Their conversation centers on matters of ontology and how ontology relates to thinking about disability.

Ontology is thought to play a central role within disabilities ethics. In this formulation, what something *is* determines the obligations owed it. Accordingly, ontology concerns itself with what things *are* and by extension the obligations that follow. We might determine, for instance, that X is ontologically human (say, possesses human qualities) but distinguish between humans and persons where the distinction makes the moral difference of claiming obligations for one and not the other. This formulation finds an analogy in a classic defense of abortion rights where Mary Anne Warren distinguishes between persons and human fetuses, where the rights of the mother as person supersede the rights of the fetus as human.[1] Warren goes on to specify the conditions by which humans become persons—i.e., namely when possessed of consciousness, reasoning, self-motivated activity, communicative capacities, and self-awareness—such that human fetuses are at most potential persons whereas mothers are actual persons. Warren's specifications are meant to be applied, insofar as they are ontological specifications about personhood, to other cases where personhood comes into question, with obvious implications for disability ethics. If one's disability means one no longer meets the conditions of personhood (i.e., one no longer possesses the ability to reason, communicate, etc.), then is one still owed the rights of persons? Indeed, the disabled turn out to serve as counterexamples to Warren's formulation since few would endorse taking rights away from the disabled because of their disabilities.[2] However one feels about Warren's argument about fetuses as nonpersons, her formulation proves illustrative of how ontological status (e.g., "Is X a person or merely human?") becomes a common point of departure for a wide range of moral questions including disability. Theology gets brought into the ontological formulation once it is thought that theology definitively tells us what anything is (i.e., what some thing is to God tells us what that thing is definitively). For example, one might claim the disabled as specially bearing God's image in a way that morally obligates us toward them regardless of their status as persons.

In the following, Tran and Bishop discuss the question of whether ontology should play the role granted by the formulation. Tran starts off by arguing that beginning with ontology (i.e., taking the question of personhood as one's analytical point of departure on questions of disability) does not get us very far. Tran argues instead for an account of moral reflection where ontology comes later, if at all. Bishop is not so sure. While he agrees with Tran that modern conversations exaggerate and overinterpret the role of ontology, he thinks the relationship between ontology and moral action is closer than Tran admits, and the intimacy of that relationship is part of what grants creaturely life its moral salience. Dispensing with certain terminological differences, the conversation then turns to this intimacy and its importance for moral life, and how Christianity does or does not make good on it in how it imagines the disabled.

Jonathan Tran: It is often assumed in bioethics generally and disability studies particularly that ethical questions depend on ontological questions. The idea here is that how a person is treated depends on how she is categorized ontologically—namely, whether her human status is sufficiently established to secure human treatment.[3] If she is seen as human, she will be treated humanely (i.e., how a human being should be treated). The formulation, which we can call the ontological formula, can be summarized as human treatment. In other words, anyone whom we call a human person should receive humane treatment. Coming under the heading of ontology (ontology concerning itself with *being*, i.e., what some thing *is*), the formula regularly shows up in discussions about abortion, stem cell research, and cloning, in turn leading to furious debates about who counts as what.[4] Is the fetus a person in the same way the mother is a person? Questions of personhood also arise within conversations about disability. Insofar as some think what makes humans distinct from other animals is their rational minds, one could discount the personhood of those whose rational capacities have been disabled. The problem disability accordingly presents then has everything to do with how rights depend on abilities just as abilities depend on personhood. The work of the ethicist committed to disability rights then amounts to the work of securing rights even when abilities have diminished and personhood has come into question. "Even if she cannot X, Y, and Z, she's still a person and so should be treated as such" is what the appeal looks like. As Romero and Eberl argue in chapter 3, Christian theologians such as Aquinas adopted a theologically informed version of this ontological formula. A person's status as a person serves as the ultimate trump card, with her rights held as inviolable irrespective of ability.

Notice two things about the ontological formula. First is how it trades in abstractions about persons as such rather than dealing with the concrete realities through which persons come to matter in the first place. The claim "Even if she cannot X, Y, and Z, she's still a person" proceeds as if "person" so defines itself that its mere invocation wins the argument. The thought is that once personhood is established (once we get our ontology straight), then the matter is settled. To get a sense of the formula's abstract nature, contrast "Even if she cannot X, Y, and Z, she's still a person" with "Even if Aunty Lien cannot X, Y, and Z, I still love her."[5] Aunty Lien and my feelings for her are not abstract but concrete—carrying as they do conceptual, narrative, and practical force—such that X, Y, and Z (and their loss) mean what they do in the context of our relationship. Not only is the ontological formula thought to carry weight independent of these conceptual, narrative, and practical realities, but its power comes in its ability to do so, as an appeal that can be made devoid of relational commitments, a word spoken to strangers (i.e., those about whom little can be conceptually, narratively, or practically assumed). I will return to this later.

Notice secondly that insomuch as the formula grants "human being" enough ontological weight to warrant humane treatment, it comes with the implication that those considered less than human warrant less moral consideration. If ontological status matters most and human status trumps all, then a lesser ontological status means less moral consideration. "Less" might mean no more than "less than the moral consideration accorded to humans," but still a calculus of more and less obtains. I will return to this as well.

Against the ontological formula, I think that when it comes to bioethics and disability studies, ontological assertions do little work, and, when they actually do something, they do so on the back end. Ordinary claims of the kind that actually order our moral lives (e.g., "Even if Aunty Lien cannot X, Y, and Z, I still love her") do not begin with ontological appeals followed by practical applications (i.e., "human" humane treatment). Rather, ontology sits in the background of practical arrangements and helps make sense of them when such help is needed, which is rare enough. Two things go into this. First is a distinction between justifying a claim and grounding it.[6] Justifying a claim entails squaring an action so that it is consistent with accepted norms of behavior.[7] Showing how that action coheres with "how we do things around here" works well enough in most cases.[8] My actions are justified insofar as they prove continuous with all our actions. Ontology plays no role at this juncture. Justifying a claim (e.g., "that action is good") requires no court of appeals beyond us (e.g., we deem such actions good). Now, ontological appeals can, when needed (say, when talking to strangers—those not counted as "us"), ground such claims beyond us (where grounding describes—which is not to say, justifies—what I perceive to be a basis beyond us), but, importantly, not in a way that takes over the justifying function. Those who subscribe to the ontological formula confuse the justifying and grounding functions, underestimating the former and overinterpreting the latter. The operative norms of behavior in which my life with Aunty Lien unfolds—which issue from the concepts through which I relate to her, the narratives by which I frame our relationship, and the practical projects that make her "my Aunty Lien"—will prove sufficient for justifying my claim that she ought to be treated as someone I love.[9] To be sure, any relationship can go any number of ways—that is, "Even if Aunty Lien can X, Y, and Z, I still hate her" is as possible as "Even if Aunty Lien cannot X, Y, and Z, I still love her." How I relate to her diminished X, Y, and Z will largely depend on how I relate to her generally. If my life's practical projects can include her diminished X, Y, and Z, then her incapacities will matter that much less and it will not occur to me to love her differently. If the story that frames our shared lives, as another criterion of judgment, requires her X, Y, and Z, then I will have a harder time adjusting to our new situation. And if the concepts through which I envision our life together depend on her possessing X, Y, and Z, then things will go still another way. My life with her before she loses X, Y, and Z for the most part determines my life with her after she loses them. If after she loses X, Y, and Z, I begin to treat her inhumanely, it will indicate not that I have judged her less than human and acted accordingly but that I did not love her as I claimed (say, unconditionally). The discovery will be not her inhumanness but rather my inhumanity.

The same can be said regarding a baby who is born to me without the possibility of X, Y, and Z. How I relate to him largely depends on how I already relate to him. If he is born without the possibility of X, Y, and Z, then it will not suddenly occur to me due to some ontological belief that what I now have in front of me is something less than my child. His disability will not put me down a path of wondering about his personhood. What will matter is how I relate to him as mine, someone whose life makes demands on my life, or not.[10] Indeed, should I begin to refer to Aunty Lien or my newborn baby as "a human being," that itself will indicate something has gone wrong, not with her or him but with me. Similarly, no one when forced to euthanize her dog actually consoles herself with "Well, Fido is just a dog." At no point in Fido's life, even and especially at the end, does she relate to him on ontological grounds.[11]

There might be occasions where I need to ground my judgment about Aunty Lien or Fido by invoking ontological appeals—"She's a human being" or "He's only a dog"—but such occasions are not only rare but often perverse, and it is unclear to whom other than strangers such appeals are made. If anything, appeals of that sort are usually made to license *inhumane* treatment, and one wonders if such instances are the real purpose of the ontological formula, as ideological justification for problematic behavior.[12] It might be the case that moral life is now so bereft of ethical substance that the best we can do is appeal to strangers using blanket claims about personhood. But such a state of affairs only further demonstrates the poverty of ontological appeals (as will be demonstrated later in reference to the philosopher Peter Singer).

Jeffrey Bishop: I find most of what you, Tran, have written to be right, though I might frame it differently. I agree that ontological appeals are impoverished, especially when they are garnered to do positive work, whether that work be to permit behaviors like justifying the use of certain people for experimentation, or the appeal to ontological categories to leverage forms of protection for those that might be experimented upon.

I wonder if what you have written overly reifies the distinction between praxis and theory. The practical emerges in the world of narrative and emotion; certainly, that is correct. And the ontological emerges from the realm of theory, abstraction, analysis, and definition. Yet, I would argue that embedded in any form of action—practical or theoretical—there are already ontological assumptions that are active, even if in a nonconscious way. The theoretical carries the practical with it; practice carries theory with it. The latter means that ontological abstractions are part of what animates practical activity, something Pryor in Chapter 1 similarly argues regarding transhumanism.

I think I would prefer to see the interlacing of the practical and theoretical, and point to a prior distinction between analysis and intuition, following Henri Bergson.[13] Both the practical and the theoretical emerge from the activities of intellect. For Bergson, the primary activities of intellect are analysis and intuition, and each is active in theoretical work and in practical work. Analysis is at work in the doing of science as well as in the doing of metaphysics in the contemporary sense of the word. I think by focusing on these two activities—analysis and intuition—we might come closer to seeing that within the practical activity of the scientist (the doing of science or metaphysics) and the practical activities of those who love Aunty Lien or Fido (the taking care of Aunty Lien or Fido), there are embedded ontological assumptions. For example, on the side of the practical, one sees the ontological assumptions built into practical activity when one asks the question, "Why have you sent Fido outside to relieve his bladder or his bowels instead of showing him to the hall powder room?" In walking to the door to let Fido out, one is not actively considering the ontological categories. But they are none-theless active. Why does one show Fido outside but show Aunty Lien to the hall toilet? The fact that these ontological categories are non-conscious does not mean that they are not active.

In the practical work of the scientist, theories—which are post hoc reconstructions after analysis—are also operative nonconsciously. From the side of theory, I think we can agree that the supposed theo-retical work of scientists or metaphysicians, or those who would want to deploy ontological categories, are actually governed by pragmatic concerns.[14] I think most scientific theories are built out of pragmatic concerns, whether those practical concerns are focused on getting experiments to work, or getting the ideas to conform to multiple data points, or trying to get multiple data points derived from method-ologically distinct approaches to align. Theory reconstructs the world after analysis has cut (ana–lysis, lysed, cut) the world of things into parts that had been wholes. That cutting can be the literal cutting with the scalpel or the cutting by the scalpel–like mind.[15]

Put differently, I would say, with Henri Bergson, that the work of analysis (science and metaphysics) is part of the mythmaking activ-ity of intellect as much as intuition is.[16] When engaged in analy-sis, one is in the process of cutting the world into bits, and, after cutting it into bits, one has to reconstruct those bits into imagi-native wholes—that is, construct theories, construct myths to put the pieces back together. So analysis is engaged with parts (parts that have been created by the lysis of the intellect), and it must reconstruct them into wholes. Intuition guides one in reconstruct-ing the wholes but recognizes that wholes precede the cutting work of analysis. Intuition also recognizes that theories are insufficient to account for the whole. Yet, intuition also emerges from our having been cultivated historically by the historical working out of "theory and practice," founded upon the prior work that analysis has done.

So, I would want to blur the lines between theory and practice, and say that there is a continuity between these two domains; the problem arises prior to the theoretical and practical distinction. Moreover, I would say that the distinction between theory and prac-tice is already the artifice created by analysis. In fact, there is a kind of

everydayness about scientific, analytic, abstract language of ontology, but there is also a thicker ontological set of commitments in the
everyday, emotional, narratival language of love for Aunty Lien. For
those living life with Aunty Lien, and laughing with her, caring for her,
being cared for by her, and so on, one does not appeal to ontological,
abstract, scientific language, but even in the everyday language there
is a "folk" ontology at work. The folk ontology is at work in the everyday care offered to Aunty Lien. One only makes the ontology explicit
if someone is asked, as Peter Singer asked of Eva Kittay about Sesha,
whether Sesha's psychological properties were akin to those of a pig.[17]

Here, then, is the crux of the matter. Singer's question fundamentally disrupts the folk ontology at work in the everyday care that
Kittay gives to Sesha; but then Singer's question emerges from his
own "folk" ontology, which he thinks somehow has greater purchase
as "true," even while it is the artifice of a prior analysis. Singer's "folk"
ontology is a post hoc reconstruction that arises out of the analysis
done by the long history of positivism and British empiricism. For
unclear reasons, the late modern, majority culture grants this ontology pride of place, and proclaims it to be "true." The natural reaction
is for Kittay to defend her "folk" ontology already at work in the care
that she gives her daughter. Kittay delights in the delight that Sesha
takes from playing music for example, but she plays music because
she knows that Sesha enjoys music, that Sesha is the kind of being
that can enjoy music.

What distinguishes the two ontologies—Kittay's and
Singer's—then, may not be the philosophical analysis of pigs and
Sesha, or Fido and Aunty Lien, but rather the work that one is hoping to do, or is expecting to have to do with the language. But the
"theoretical" carries a practical dimension, and the "practical" carries
a theoretical dimension. On the "folk" ontology at work in Singer's
question, the practical dimension falls into the background as the
scientist/metaphysician makes claims—builds myths—about the
nature of a thing, eliding the practical that informs his definition. On
the "folk" ontology already at work in Kittay's love for Sesha and Tran's
love of Aunty Lien—and my love for Sesha and Aunty Lien, because I
trust Kittay and Tran, much more than I trust Singer—there is a "theoretical" dimension that falls into the background of the practical work
that one hopes to do in offering that love. After all, Kittay and Tran

have an intuition that Sesha and Aunty Lien are wholes that resist the reductive categorizations offered by Singer, even if Singer—his thinking obscured by his analysis and his mythologies—occludes the intuition from even occurring to him.

What you are asking is that we do not fall into the trap of a different kind of analysis and subsequent mythologizing in response to those that have ontologized Sesha and pigs into the same sort of categories. After all, all ontological claims—like all scientific claims—will ultimately fall short of beings like Sesha and Aunty Lien, and pigs and Fido, because they are an artifice of our theorizing/ontologizing. But the problem is that the human intellect is always engaged in analysis and intuition, and the process of mythmaking is the fine balancing act that we are always engaged in as human actors. That sounds scary because the human seems to need rock solid ground on which to stand. However, all ontological claims are ultimately historical, political, and practical in orientation, even if we say they are theoretical claims.

But to resign ourselves to the fact that all our theoretical categorizations are handed to us historically, politically, and practically is to admit we stand on shaky ground, and it worries us that the shaky ground might result in our putting Sesha and Aunty Lien into categories with pigs instead of with persons. Our worry is that upon such a shaky ground, others who do not love Sesha and Aunty Lien the way we do might miss the point that beings like Sesha and Aunty Lien may come to be imagined as indistinct from pigs and Fido. But we must also remember that Sesha and Aunty Lien, as well as pigs and Fido, as living being are far in excess of our theories or ontologies. Whether Singer's pig quip or Kittay's ontologizing, each stands outside all the ontological reductions—whether Singer's folk ontology or Kittay's.

So, I would argue that our mistake is that we prefer ossified ontologies, which are post hoc reconstructions that are necessary because of *pre hoc* analysis. As my colleague Kimbell Kornu has pointed out, we live in the age of a dissective rationality, a dissective rationality that has suffused the West. Our tendency, especially where science and contemporary metaphysics reign, is to valorize analysis—to valorize the cutting of the world into parts. Once it is cut into parts through the artifice of rationality, we must once again reconstruct the parts into an artificial whole; but existing wholes like

Sesha and Aunty Lien resist being cut into artificial parts to begin with and the mechanical reconstructions that need follow the cutting. Put differently, Sesha and Aunty Lien are in excess of the cuts deployed by Singer and by analytic metaphysicians who would try to save them from Singer's dissection.

So, from whence shall come our salvation from analytic, dissective rationality, from the ontologizing stupor created by late modern analysis? I want to argue that our attunement has to move more toward the cultivation of intuition in excess of analysis. One has an intuition that Singer is wrong (and Singer has trained himself out of the practices of intuition), because in taking up with Sesha or Aunty Lien, or pigs or Fido, one has the intuition that, whatever parsed reconstructions we engage in, the beings that are Sesha, Aunty Lien, pigs, and Fido resist our ontologizing categorizations. They even resist the categorizations that would put pigs and Sesha into the same category. We have a deep, felt sense that the whole that is Aunty Lien is far in excess of what we can imagine. Aunty Lien is the gratuitous excess that saturates all of our activities of taking up with her.

Finally, what is necessary is not a better ontology or set of categories but instead the cultivation of attunement to the excess, the things that cannot be categorized, which the analytic attitude now defiantly resists. The cultivation of attunement to the excess is the cultivation of intuition, which is present and active in human life but which we have trained ourselves into not trusting. Liturgy is the practice of cultivation of intuition, which is also attunement to the excess that is Aunty Lien and Sesha. In the realm of the Christian church, the church through her liturgical activities (such as the halting movement more deeply from word to sacrament toward the mystery of faith, the recitation of the creed, the praying of the Lord's Prayer) articulates the doctrines of Trinity, incarnation, and creation.[18] At the heart of each of these doctrines is an irreducible openness to the excess, and, through the liturgy of the church, we begin to embody our practices of attunement to the excess of beings and the whole of being, and God.

If Christians reductively deploy—as we have at times in the past—our doctrines, such that they are ossified categories of Trinity or incarnation, or if creation becomes the ossified reductive category of nature, then we fall into the same problematic as Singer. So, the activity of liturgy is our own participation in the activity of

God, the activity of the incarnation, and the activity of creation. In participating in the liturgy, which is to participate in the activity of God's creating and redeeming of creation, we may then take up with God's creatures, which is the activity of taking care of Sesha and Aunty Lien. And when we must act into the unknown and unfolding of the excess that is creation, we must bow the head, for what we are doing might cut deeply into beings.

Tran: I agree with you that practice entails theory. I just want to say that theory consists of more than ontology, and particularly ontological beliefs about human status. Hence, my distinction between justifying and grounding. Justifying involves norms—that is, social practices, which are theory-laden (more on this in a moment). Grounding involves ontology—specifically, for this occasion, metaphysical categories by which one determines human status. In ordinary life, answering the question you pose ("Why have you sent Fido outside to relieve his bladder or his bowels instead of showing him to the hall powder room?") will take some version of the answer, "Because that's what we do" rather than "Because Fido is a dog." More precisely, what one's answer can mean by the latter requires something like the former: "Because that's what we do with those we *call* 'dogs.'" Words like "dog" or "Auntie Lien" come as agreements in language that provide their own justifications insofar as one speaks the language—my use is justified by speaking as others do.[19] Language, with these built-in justifications, is theory-laden in this way and therefore is well positioned to illuminate the intrinsic relationship between theory and practice as you quite rightly highlight (for me, studying how language ordinarily works reveals where and how ontology comes into play, and hence my conviction that ontology comes in on the back side, if at all).[20] This all comes under the aegis of practical reason, and practical reason involves theories that guide, interpret, and describe action and that ordinarily carry on without speculative beliefs beyond and about the action. Such beliefs, which include ontological beliefs about human categories and status, then have little direct bearing on ordinary moral activity.

So we agree that theory and practice go together but disagree on what theory entails, where you insist that it includes in some form or fashion determinative ontological commitments and I insist that theory can function without them. I think that an ordinary language account of moral action and justification suffices to show that the role moral theorists often ascribe to ontology is exaggerated and overinterpreted. Of course, those who insist on that role usually feel dissatisfied with my language-based account. For them, the problem is usually of two kinds, either that ordinary language requires ontology in ways I fail to acknowledge or that the reality of multiple languages does acknowledge this. Both of those considerations fall under what I described earlier as matters relating to conversing with strangers, and so fall outside the province of our most serious moral conversations (here, "serious" stands in for "substantive," and "substantive" presumes sharing enough narratives, concepts, and practical projects to be considered "serious").

Where we interestingly converge is on the role of the moral formation in communal, for me, concepts and, for you, intuitions.[21] Hence I share your impression of Peter Singer's philosophical project, both of us believing that one should avoid his kind of preference utilitarian analysis, since, as you say, in the ordinary case, "Kittay and Tran have an intuition that Sesha and Aunty Lien are wholes that resist the reductive categorizations offered by Singer, even if Singer—his thinking obscured by his analysis and his mythologies—occludes the intuition from even occurring to him." What Singer seems to worry about is precisely the intuitions you highlight as guiding moral action. You and I are in agreement that our lives with others before we cut them up determines whether or not we cut them up, say, as human and nonhuman animals—literally or analytically. We seem to grant moral intuitions a determinative role in a way that makes their formation crucial for us and that formation illegible (and, when legible, threatening) for the likes of Singer.

So let me end with a few comments about moral intuitions and their formation as they relate to our lives with the disabled. You say, quite evocatively, "The cultivation of attunement to the excess is the cultivation of intuition, which is present and active in human life but which we have trained ourselves into not trusting." Here you talk about that which exceeds our analytical categories, and you specifically mention those whose otherness exceeds our categorizations and our reductive tendencies toward them (e.g., "the disabled" as an ontological term of art meant to ideologically justify certain attitudes and actions). Relatedly, you worry that the kind of analysis we philosophically employ to bring the world into focus usually obscures it, and you additionally worry that, for folks like Singer, that is somewhat the point, to keep us from the world precisely because its excess would otherwise overwhelm us.

I view Singer similarly, that the too-easy categorizations presumed in his case against "speciesism" deflects something important. He wants to claim that the similarity between us and self-aware nonhuman animals means that we owe them greater moral respect than we tend to give them (the latter point seems obvious, though its obviousness does not, for me, require the ontological premise Singer sets up). He infamously pushes what he takes to be a corresponding claim, that non-self-aware humans (i.e., those with significantly diminished capacities) deserve less respect than we are inclined to give them. "Speciesism" accordingly names for him an unjust moral bias in favor of human disability on the one hand and against non-human animal ability on the other.[22] You and I disagree with him. And our collective disagreement has to do with how we approach the question. For us, the heart of the matter comes down not to relative similarities and abilities and their categorizations (all availed by certain modes of analysis) but rather to that which exceeds such categorizations (and therefore those modes of analysis). In other words, we agree that what should matter about others is not principally their similarity to us (couched often in their ability to do the kinds of things "able-bodied" humans do) but rather the many differences that separate us from them, evoking in us, drawing in here what the philosopher Cora Diamond says about non-human animal life, "a sense of the astonishment and incomprehension that there should be beings so like us, so unlike us, so astonishingly capable of being companions of ours and so unfathomably distant."[23] You then talk elegantly about intuitions that avail us to this excess—without which we incline toward sameness and its perpetuity—and about the kinds of moral formation that in turn habituate those intuitions and their availability to the otherness of the world, what you call "the cultivation of attunement to the excess." You think we need both these intuitions and trust in them, each of which requires inculcation into forms of life we consider, for that reason, virtuous.

You then proceed to offer an example of how liturgical inculcation into creedal claims regarding Trinity, incarnation, and creation can—as with inculcation into life with any set of concepts—go wrong, namely by cutting the world up into reductive ("dissective") categories. I take you to mean that we can hold Trinity, incarnation, and creation in ways that avail us to the world's excess or close us off from it. An example of availability is holding those three concepts together in ways that simultaneously confirm God's presence in the world without that presence endorsing whatever humans have made of God's world.[24] In this instance, individuals look for God, presuming enough continuity for such looking to make sense, and look for God beyond the usual places, presuming enough discontinuity for such looking to make sense. The opposite of availability would be marshalling those terms in ways that preclude either looking at all ("equivocity of being" in scholastic terms) or only looking at ourselves or simulacra of ourselves ("univocity of being" in scholastic terms).[25] Life with the disabled—those who confirm God's presence in the world without that presence endorsing whatever humans have made of God's world—then attunes us (and them) to looking, helps us trust what we find, and thereby helps us see God, what I have tried to describe as ontology coming on the back side.

Bishop: If there is a difference between what we each are saying, I hope it is only one of emphasis, as I found myself saying "Amen!" to what you have written. Ontology is the post hoc reconstruction of that which the mind has analytically cut into parts. Ontology does come in on the back side. I also suppose it becomes important to ask: Why does ontology come in at all? And then, the question is, are these post hoc ontological constructions just mistakes of a rather overconfident rational mind? Certainly, this question could be answered affirmatively, but I do not believe it is *just* a mistake of the human mind to engage in the activity of constructing post hoc ontologies. And then, another question arises: If there are these post hoc ontologies, what sort of work do they do, even if one decides they ought to do no work at all? I guess I hold that post hoc ontological constructions do some sort of work for us and are not merely mistakes, mistaken though they may be.

I will give tentative answers to these three questions: Why do ontologies come in at all? Second, if they come to do work, is it a mistake to engage in ontological constructions? And third, what is the work of ontology, and what are its limits? As much as it irks me to admit it, ontologies come along because they are indeed helpful. As a medical doctor, I have seen that these post hoc ontological reconstructions are helpful, and they are also harmful.

I will need to draw on an example in order to make the case that ontological constructions—made on the back side as they are—are still helpful. As noted by Bergson, reality is in motion, unfolding. It is in a process of becoming. Things like rocks appear to be more stable; they seem to have staying power, even as other elements of reality, wind and water, rail against them. Living beings—like ourselves—seem to have less staying power than a rock and seem to be in a dynamic relationship with their surroundings. I would call these more stable, living beings "dynamic stabilities." Relative to the flow of reality, living entities seem to persist in the chaotic flow of reality around them. They seem to work against the flow in that they have created stable structures that permit them to resist the chaotic flow of reality that surrounds them.

The slowing down of the flow that coalesces round these living entities means there is some *thing* there that works in the midst of the flow, both against and in concert with it. I will call these slowed-down motions—which persist in the midst of the flow of reality—"structures." Structures persist in time, for a time, and even repeat themselves to maintain identity. For example, in the case of a living being, the organism repeats its structures through the process of healing. Living beings also repeat themselves across time through reproduction. In other words, the success of the organism to persist in the midst of a constant flow of change surrounding it is due to its ability to repeat its structures. If it cannot repeat its own structure, it falls out of being; it ceases to exist. Sometimes, a novelty is introduced in the flow of a chaotic reality that might disrupt the living being's ability to repeat itself, through healing or reproduction. When it fails to repeat itself, the being falls out of being. In other words, when an organism cannot overcome a problem presented by the chaotic flow of reality, if it repeats the same structure that cannot overcome the problem, it falls out of being. It dies. For example, a predator species takes advantage of the repeated structures of the prey's behavior, and if the prey keeps repeating the behavior, it goes out of existence.

Now, life finds a way around such a failure to repeat itself by freeing itself from the necessary structures. The human mind—itself a product of the structures of a living being, namely the human brain—can rise above the repeated failures in the face of some threat and find a way around the failing structure. Its freedom permits it to act where the structures just habitually repeat themselves. The mind seeks to understand the failing structures of living beings in order to find a way around the failing structures of human beings. For example, a bacterium takes up residence inside the lung, hoping to exploit the rich oxygen-and-blood environment—exploiting the structures of the lung—but inadvertently kills its host. The human mind, in seeking to understand the biological structures (which are in motion, i.e., functions), finds a way to work around the structures by creating antibiotics. Thus, medicine is born. Medicine then attempts to understand the way the structures have tended to repeat themselves in order to help those structures to repeat themselves as they are failing in time.

The work of the mind uses symbols—whether linguistic or mathematical, or mythical, or artistic, or religious—to represent to itself the repeated structures of reality, frail and failing though those structures may be. What are symbols but the repeated structures of a culture that tend to align in a way that adequately represents a reality? The symbols structure our musings about the structures of reality, but the cultural symbols—including the mathematical symbols of science—are structures of the mind that seem to do some work but fail to themselves exhaust the reality that they hope to represent to the mind. In other words, medical science is a *logos* (word)—a logic—about *ontos*, an onto-logic representing ontic reality. The being of the structures of mind is a different kind of being than the being of the structure of entities—lungs, or brains, or bacteria. But the work of the mind can be and often is successful at permitting the human animal to repeat its being; that is to say, medicine can do work that is good at assisting the frail structures of life at sustaining themselves. It is capable of doing so by creating ontological constructions—representations —that are adequate for the purposes for which they are created.

However, these successes in medicine result in a kind of hubris of medicine, in that we take these helpful post hoc ontological constructions to fully represent all reality. Put differently, the onto-logic of medicine comes to think that its own words about reality—its own onto-logic—is fully representative of reality, indeed almost identical with it.

This onto-logic can be seen when medicine thinks it needs to fix disabled bodies according to the structures articulated by the medical mind. Or it can be seen on display when Singer says that Sesha, Aunty Lien, and a pig all hang together as the same kind of thing. Medicine's onto-logic, which is mostly the same as Western society's utilitarian onto-logic, is powerful in that it can and does do work; but it is also the danger of any onto-logic to think that its cultural representation—even in mathematical symbols—is adequate to the realities. Western society's scientific representation—its onto-logic—is privileged over other onto-logics. This onto-logic has become the idol to which actual beings can be sacrificed, and, in Singer's case, it somehow collapses into an ought. After all, does Singer not claim that some beings perhaps ought to be sacrificed to the onto-logic in this Western utilitarian onto-logic?

Why do we construct onto-logics? Because they work for the tasks for which they are developed. Medicine works; it is good in that its onto-logic is helpful to us for our tasks—helpful, that is to say, until it is not. Ontologies are pragmatic shorthand, used by people because they are useful. Practitioners deploy them all the time. But as we both have said, they are not adequate to the fullness of beings. Like the failing biological structures, the linguistic, mathematical, artistic, and even religious structures that the human mind creates can do work for us, but they can also fail us. After all, the work of the analytic mind that parses the world is insufficient to the interrelatedness of reality. Out of these ontological successes, the mind becomes overconfident in its onto-logical structures and then deploys them on actual beings. Now imagine you have a body that does not conform to the static ontologies built by those given power in society. Now imagine that those in power hope to build what they have taken to be correct ontologies into a future in which those ontologies have pride of place.

A problem arises very starkly when we try to build or to enhance a body (abled or disabled) precisely because the onto-logic of human anatomy and physiology, while useful up to a point, extends the static onto-logical structures—products of our own time and our onto-logics—into a future as if that future is not itself active, as if that future is not a flow. Put differently, whatever the goods we imagine possible by our onto-logics, they are merely the repetitions of what we take the goods of the world to be at the time of their design. They repeat the past goods that have been normed by the onto-logics imagined at a specific time. Biologically this may not be so bad; bodies, while certainly in flux, are relatively stable in their biological structures. However, enhancement is not merely the repeated onto-logics of biological functioning. Even this biological functioning carries the social, moral, and political imaginary with it as it is deployed on the body.

Bioenhancement, then, does not deploy a future, but it enacts—literally materializes in the body—the past goods of the onto-logics regnant at the time. And insofar as those ontologies are ontologies that exclude nonconforming bodies, what gets built in the future are the old ontologies of technoscience. In repeating the goods as imagined by the present, the engineered future is doomed to a repetition of the present that has now passed and has become the past. Thus, the past exclusionary onto-logics enact the exclusionary spirit of the social, moral, and political structures of the past. It is not that enhancement is messing around with human nature—a static nature—but that it asks the bodies of the "enhanced" to repeat the imagined onto-logics of a particular limited present that always fall short of the realities of living beings.

Certainly, we create these onto-logical structures to be helpful, and they are indeed helpful. They are not mere mistakes, because they can be and in some instances have been helpful. But the onto-logics, even in their usefulness and helpfulness, will always fall short of the creatures they purport to help. They can become problematic insofar as they enact a particular social, moral, or political order, itself also a product of its time, which in time comes to ossify. Insofar as the technoscientific ontology of bodies asks all bodies to conform to them, they do violence to nonconforming bodies.

Ontologies come about because these constructions are helpful to the work of surviving in a world of frailty, up to a point. Thus, onto-logical constructions do work and are not mere mistakes, though they will always be mistaken at some level. I do not think that someone that attempts to counter the post hoc onto-logical constructions of medicine or of Peter Singer is merely making a mistake in uncovering the ontology at play in the dominant, technoscientific utilitarianism of Singer. In attempting to create alternative accounts that compete with Singer's onto-logical account of disabled bodies, one may in fact trouble the waters of Singer's account. Laying out Singer's onto-logic and asking if it conforms to our experience is in fact helpful to Auntie Lien and Sesha. So, turning to ontology to counter other ontologies can be helpful to wake a culture from its ontologizing stupor. But we must not take the competing onto-logical account to be the final account. Ontology has work to do, but it must recognize its limits.

The tendency in our onto-logical constructions—which are post hoc reconstructions of the world after the analytic mind has cut it into parts—is to assume that our cuts and our reconstructions fully represent reality without leaving an excess or a remainder. These onto-logical constructions that say that Sesha is not only like a pig, but no different from a pig, or that Aunty Lien is not only like Fido, but no different from Fido, are mistaken.

Recognizing the limits of these constructions—necessary though they may be for certain tasks—requires us to bow the head and to press pause on the analytic-reconstructive activity of the mind, to recognize the limits of any onto-logical constructions, including those that would counter Singer's onto-logic. Divine liturgy is the place where we gain the habits of suspending the analytic-reconstructing of reality, for God does not fit into our categories, doctrines, concepts, or ontologies. We mistakenly take creatures like bread and wine to be merely bread and wine under our naturalistic ontologies. Liturgy reveals to us in the gratuitous gift of creation and redemption that they are the incarnate and resurrected body and life-giving blood of Christ. Liturgy is the work of bowing the head and placing one's voice in subservient service of the Other and the other in a way that is neither univocal nor equivocal, but in a way that is in-between, participating in the activity of Trinitarian creation in and through the incarnational gift. By participating in the activity of the incarnation (of which the liturgy is itself an extension) and by taking the flesh of Christ into our own flesh, one is taken up into the activity of creation, which is the ongoing activity of the Trinity. That then is our true worship, divine liturgy. Those whom we have labeled disabled might then come to be seen as the flowing forth of creation, not its mistakes. And we come alongside these fellow creatures, or, rather, as they come alongside us, we find together we are becoming the fulfillment of creation.

Notes

1 Mary Anne Warren, "On the Moral and Legal Status of Abortion," *Monist* 57, no. 1 (1973): 43–61.

2 Francis Beckwith makes this argument in *Defending Life: A Moral and Legal Case against Abortion Choice* (New York: Cambridge University Press, 2007), 130–72.

3 Consider Bill Hughes, "Being Disabled: Towards a Critical Social Ontology for Disability Studies," *Disability & Society* 22, no. 7 (2007): 673–84; D. Christopher Ralston and Justin Ho, "Disability, Humanity, and Personhood: A Survey of Moral Concepts," *Journal of Medicine and Philosophy* 32, no. 6 (2007): 619–33; and Maayan Agmon, Amalia Sa'ar, and Tal Araten-Bergman, "The Person in the Disabled Body: A Perspective on Culture and Personhood from the Margins," *International Journal for Equity in Health* 15, no. 147 (2016): 1–12.

4 See Paul Lauritzen's rendition of the ontological formula in relationship to stem cell research and abortion in his 2003 President's Council on Bioethics paper "The Ethics of Stem Cell Research," available at https://biotech.law.lsu.edu/research/pbc/background/lauritzen_paper.html. Earlier, see H. Tristram Engelhardt, "The Ontology of Abortion," *Ethics* 84, no. 3 (1974): 217–34.

5 "Aunty Lien" is my take on Stanley Hauerwas' "Uncle Charlie" in his famous essay "Must a Patient Be a Person to Be a Patient? Or, My Uncle Charlie Is Not Much of a Person, but He Is Still My Uncle Charlie," in *The Hauerwas Reader*, ed. John Berkman and Michael G. Cartwright (Durham, N.C.: Duke University Press, 2001), 596–602.

6 I draw this distinction from John Bowlin's "Status, Ideal, and Calling: Languages of the Human," *Journal of the Society of Christian Ethics* 41, no. 2 (2021): 231–35. In developing the distinction, Bowlin references Gideon Rosen, "Metaphysical Dependence: Grounding and Reduction," in *Modality: Metaphysics, Logic, and Epistemology*, ed. Bob Hale and Aviv Hoffmann (Oxford: Oxford University Press, 2010), 109–35.

7 See Robert Brandom's delineation in *A Spirit of Trust: A Reading of Hegel's Phenomenology* (Cambridge, Mass.: Belknap Press of Harvard University Press, 2019), 22–23.

8 See Stanley Cavell's discussion in "The Availability of Wittgenstein's Later Philosophy," *Philosophical Review* 71, no. 1 (1962): 67–93 (72–74).

9 On how concepts, narratives, and projects grant normative objectivity justifying power, see Alice Crary, *Inside Ethics: On the Demands of Moral Thought* (Cambridge, Mass.: Harvard University Press, 2016), 36–91.

10 For an account of being so claimed, see Brian Brock, *Wondrously Wounded: Theology, Disability, and the Body of Christ* (Waco, Tex.: Baylor University Press, 2019).

11   For more along these lines, see Cora Diamond, "Eating Meat and Eating People," *Philosophy* 53, no. 206 (1978): 465–79.

12   I argue as much in relationship to American chattel slavery specifically and racial capitalism generally in Jonathan Tran, *Asian Americans and the Spirit of Racial Capitalism* (Oxford: Oxford University Press, 2022).

13   See especially Henri Bergson's essay "An Introduction to Metaphysics," in *The Creative Mind: An Introduction to Metaphysics*, trans. Mabelle L. Andison (Minneola, N.Y.: Dover, 2007). It should be noted that for Bergson analysis is the work of science, the activity of taking things apart and as dealing in parts that post hoc have to be reconstructed. Analysis creates an artificial stasis, and, because things are themselves in motion, the idea of analytic metaphysics would make no sense to him. Bergson has a very specific meaning for metaphysics proper, which is an activity of intuition. Intuition extends consciousness (which is itself a flow) into the flow of things. Intuition is in sympathy with the flow of beings. Intuition that is the flow of mind is the work of metaphysics, the taking up with wholes that are in themselves irreducible by the activity of analysis and stasis. Given these senses of analysis and intuition, contemporary metaphysics would be more akin to science than to Bergson's notion of metaphysics.

14   The same pragmatic concerns are also governing the deployment of ontological categories when the scientist insists on ontological differences between Aunty Lien and Fido for how to treat Aunty Lien's indigestion or Fido's. And moral pragmatics govern the ontological distinction for claiming that one ought not to put Aunty Lien outside to use the toilet.

15   Kimbell Kornu has several papers pointing out the logic of analysis, including "Anatomy of Being, Metaphysics of Death: The Case of Avicenna's Logical Dissection," *Journal of Bioethical Inquiry* 18, no. 4 (2021): 655–69; "Medical *Ersatz* Liturgies of Death: Anatomical Dissection and Organ Donation as Biopolitical Practices," *Heythrop Journal* LXIII (2022): 386–400, https://doi.org/10.1111/heyj.13574; "Enchanted Nature, Dissected Nature: The Case of Galen's Anatomical Theology," *Theoretical Medicine and Bioethics* 39, no 6 (2018): 453–71, and "Asclepius against the Crucified: Medical Nihilism and Incarnational Life in Death," *Christian Bioethics* 23, no. 1 (2017): 38–59.

16   See especially Henri Bergson, *Two Sources of Morality and Religion*, trans. R. Ashley Audra and Cloudesley Bereton (Notre Dame: University of Notre Dame Press, 1977 [1932]).

17   Eva Feder Kittay, "The Personal Is Philosophical Is Political: A Philosopher and Mother of a Cognitively Disabled Person Sends Notes from the Battlefield," *Metaphilosophy* 40, nos. 3–4 (2009): 606–27 (621).

18   It is also true that these doctrines themselves can become reductive and indeed have become reductive in history, permitting Christian violence in many instances. If these doctrines are taken to exist outside of the lived practice of liturgy, where Trinity, incarnation, and creation are encounters, then the church falters.

19   Stanley Cavell, *The Claim of Reason: Wittgenstein, Skepticism, Morality, and Tragedy* (New York: Oxford University Press, 1979), 52.

20   For a fuller account, see my "Linguistic Theology: Completing Postliberalism's Linguistic Task," *Modern Theology* 33, no. 1 (2017), 47–68.

21   For something similar, see Julius Kovesi, *Moral Notions* (London: Routledge & Kegan Paul, 1967).

22   See, for example, his account of "self-awareness," in Peter Singer, *Animal Liberation* (New York: New York Review, 1975), 54. See Cora Diamond's critique of Singer's locution "even a retarded human being," in *The Realistic Spirit: Wittgenstein, Philosophy, and the Mind* (Cambridge, Mass.: MIT Press, 1995), 23.

23   Cora Diamond, "The Difficulty of Reality and the Difficulty of Philosophy," *Journal of Literature and the History of Ideas* 1, no. 2 (June 2003): 1–26. Also see the exchange between Diamond and Cavell, in Stanley Cavell, Cora Diamond, John McDowell, Ian Hacking, and Cary Wolfe, *Philosophy and Animal Life* (New York: Columbia University Press, 2008), 43–126.

24   Here, one might imagine a position between two kinds of Trinitarianism, that of Sarah Coakley's *God, Sexuality, and the Self: An Essay "On the Trinity"* (Cambridge: Cambridge University Press, 2013) and that of Linn Marie Tonstad's *God and Difference: The Trinity, Sexuality, and the Transformation of Finitude* (New York: Routledge, 2016).

25   See Przywara's account in Erich Przywara, *Analogia Entis: Metaphysics; Original Structure and Universal Rhythm*, trans. John Betz and David Bentley Hart (Grand Rapids: Eerdmans, 2014). See also Betz' "Beyond the Sublime: The Aesthetics of the Analogy of Being (Part One)," *Modern Theology* 21, no. 3 (2005): 367–411; and "Beyond the Sublime: The Aesthetics of the Analogy of Being (Part Two)," *Modern Theology* 22, no. 1 (2006): 1–50.

II
TRANSFIGURING VULNERABILITY

5

TRANSFIGURING THE VULNERABILITY OF SUFFERING

Kimbell Kornu

As a palliative care physician, I regard two fundamental aspects of my medical vocation to be relieving suffering and comforting the dying. I have witnessed a variety of extreme suffering: from families arguing with each other as the patient screams out in pain, to a patient yelling obscenities at his daughter because of confused agitation, to the family waiting for a seeming eternity for the patient to die after withdrawal of mechanical ventilation, to a patient begging me to hasten their death because they cannot bear the suffering of continued life. These patients and their families are some of the most vulnerable among us. They are at the mercy of the medical teams to attend to their suffering. Unfortunately, some medical teams functionally abandon their patients who are "going to die anyway" because "nothing more can be done" (from a curative standpoint). From this medicalized perspective, "doing something" means *cure*. But in my experience, attending to the suffering of patients and families requires a fuller kind of "doing"—the work of compassion, literally "suffering with." Suffering persons must be heard and comforted. And in order to do so, one must enter into that suffering with the person. Based on Matthew 25, Christ is found among those who suffer from poverty, sickness, and imprisonment. Doing the work of compassion is to serve and to suffer with the suffering Christ. In this way, suffering with can be a divine mode of existence.

Transhumanism would just as well eliminate suffering altogether. How does the transhumanist movement understand itself? At its heart, transhumanism explicitly seeks to go beyond the human.[1] Transhumanists assume that religion has traditionally provided immortality, bliss, and godlike intelligence, but now it is possible to attain these things through technology. Humanity+ (the transhumanist organization that publishes the Transhumanist Declaration, the Transhumanist Manifesto, and the Transhumanist FAQ) formally defines "transhumanism" in two parts:

(1) The intellectual and cultural movement that affirms the possibility and desirability of fundamentally improving the human condition through applied reason, especially by developing and making widely available technologies to eliminate aging and to greatly enhance human intellectual, physical, and psychological capacities.

(2) The study of the ramifications, promises, and potential dangers of technologies that will enable us to overcome fundamental human limitations, and the related study of the ethical matters involved in developing and using such technologies.[2]

A key assumption in the transhumanist project of improving the human condition is overcoming suffering. For Max More, one of the founders of the movement, transhumanism seeks to exceed the limitations of human nature that are not desirable such as suffering and death.[3] Likewise, for Nick Bostrom, human enhancement entails the continued widespread alleviation of suffering and the ideal of the "elimination of unnecessary suffering."[4] However, More admits that transhumanism cannot overcome all suffering: even if disease, aging, and death are overcome, humans will still harm, attack, and eliminate one another.[5] In response, bioethicists such as Julian Savulescu call for technologies that enhance our morality to ensure that civilization does not destroy itself.[6] In all cases, transhumanists agree that suffering is evil and must be overcome. Because suffering stems from human limitations and finitude, transhumanists exalt will, power, and the individual self.

A number of theologians find an affinity between transhumanism and Christianity in the doctrine of deification. They draw on the frequent observation that transhumanism is already a kind of auto-deification through technological modification of the human to exceed the human. Ronald Cole-Turner argues provocatively that "transhumanism" is a fundamentally Christian concept, tracing the idea back to Dante in the term *transmanar*, precisely because of theosis. He compares transhumanism and Christianity as two different means of deification: the former by technology and the latter by grace. Cole-Turner sees technology as a proper way for humans to contribute to the transformation of humans and creation, as long as one grants that it is ultimately God's work. Christ is the purpose of Christian transhumanism because humanity and all of creation are brought into transfiguration.[7] Cole-Turner problematically conflates transformation, transfiguration, and transhumanization, blurring important distinctions about deification, especially between the means of technology and the means of grace.

King-Ho Leung explores the "meta-theological" implications of deification by technology and deification by grace. He argues that Aquinas' conception of nature and grace helps us understand their relation. Drawing on the Thomistic distinction between healing grace and elevating grace, Leung provides correlations between grace in a Christian theological framework and technology in a medical-technological framework: healing grace is akin to therapy, elevating grace to enhancement, and deifying grace to transhumanism. In this schema, transhumanist technology is a form of secular grace that removes human corruptibility. However, Leung cautions that the theologization of technology can dangerously and unwittingly become a technologization of theology.[8] Leung's meta-theological framework shows how Cole-Turner falls into the trap of assuming a technological imaginary for understanding grace.

Others who are more critical of transhumanism have affirmed creatureliness and even cruciformity[9] as essential to human life, but none have specifically taken up the problem of suffering. But we must. The two kinds of deification on offer are not the same. Rather than look for a way around human suffering as the transhumanists do, Christianity points the way through it. The Epistle to the Hebrews is clear on this point, using the language of painful discipline from a father to a son:

And have you forgotten the exhortation that addresses you as sons?

"My son, do not regard lightly the discipline of the Lord,
nor be weary when reproved by him.
For the Lord disciplines the one he loves, and chastises
every son whom he receives."

It is for discipline that you have to endure. God is treating you as sons. For what son is there whom his father does not discipline? If you are left without discipline, in which all have participated, then you are illegitimate children and not sons. Besides this, we have had earthly fathers who disciplined us and we respected them. . . . For the moment all discipline seems painful rather than pleasant, but later it yields the peaceful fruit of righteousness to those who have been trained by it. (Heb 12:5–9, 11, ESV)

The Christian tradition has interpreted this passage to mean that suffering can be beneficial to one's growth as sons and daughters of God. Thus, a Christian theological engagement with transhumanism and deification needs to confront the issue of suffering. The key to understanding is Christ, the archetypal human, who "although he was a son, he learned obedience through what he suffered" (Heb 5:8, ESV) unto divine filiation.[10] In this chapter, I argue that the grace of deification is accomplished in union with Christ, in part, by way of suffering unto divine filiation. Deification entails going beyond the human to become divine, while paradoxically remaining essentially human. Consequently, suffering is transfigured: suffering, not technological bioenhancement, is the way to true human enhancement.

The argument proceeds as follows. First, I explore how the grace of deification is accomplished through suffering, looking at Maximus the Confessor's discussion of the two wills of Christ and Christ's suffering in Gethsemane. Christ in Gethsemane expresses the fulfillment of divine filiation, upon the complete alignment of Christ's human will with the divine will. Second, I examine deification in light of Luther's *theologia crucis* and how suffering is a kind of "Christosis." A human's divine mode of existing is filial and cruciform and thus Christoform. Third, I look at deification and Augustine's *totus Christus*, on how the church as the body of Christ is transfigured into the form of Christ the Head. The church is Christoform as the members of the body suffer with one another in compassion. Taken together, deification through suffering unto divine filiation critiques transhumanism in three ways: Maximus' two wills of Christ critique transhumanist exaltation of the will, Luther's *theologia crucis* critiques transhumanist power ontology, and Augustine's *totus Christus* critiques transhumanist individualism. I conclude that suffering is a means to true human enhancement: transfiguration, not transhumanism, is the proper paradigm to suffering.

Before proceeding, I want to make three clarifications. For the purposes of this chapter, I assume that "deification," "divinization," and "theosis" are synonymous terms. Second, I assume that suffering is not an intrinsic good. Suffering is a consequence of the fall and is not something to be desired in itself. Part of the healing vocation of medicine is the relief of suffering. Suffering is not the content of deification; indeed, the eschatological fulfillment of deification entails the eradication of suffering. Third, medical interventions for the relief of suffering are not necessarily opposed to the spiritual benefits of suffering. Allowing someone to suffer when there are pharmacological interventions such as analgesics that are noninvasive, efficacious, and readily available could be a form of willful negligence that worsens one's spiritual condition. However, there are instances when suffering cannot be mitigated by medical means alone without eliminating the sufferer.[11] Palliative care patients can still suffer psychologically and emotionally even with the best medical pain regimen. This chapter is intended to provide a theological framework for those who continue to suffer and for those who suffer with them in order to see how suffering can enhance, not worsen, their spiritual condition.

MAXIMUS THE CONFESSOR ON DEIFICATION AND THE WILL

The Transhumanist Declaration is a succinct document that distills core transhumanist values. Proposition 8 states: "We favour allowing individuals wide personal choice over how they enable their lives."[12] There is an unspoken assumption that the inability to

have complete personal choice in how one lives one's life, including whether one inhabits a biologically human body or some other
material substrate, can be a source of suffering due to inability
to actualize one's desire. In other words, the inability to exercise
the will to fulfill one's desire results in suffering. But this is not
the Christian account of suffering. If anything, it is its opposite. In
this section, we will explore the importance of Maximus the Confessor's elucidation of the two wills of Christ with a view toward
understanding suffering over against the exaltation of the will in
transhumanism.

Christology reveals the proper way to be human. In *Christ the
Heart of Creation*, Rowan Williams develops the sweeping thesis that
the logic of Christology illuminates the logic of the relation between
Creator and creation, and thus the logic of the relation between God
and human.[13] Christology is the key to the logic of creation because
Christ is the "perfectly creaturely."[14] But when studying the logic of
Christology, one encounters a multitude of paradoxes, notably the
relation between the infinite and the finite. Williams argues that the
paradox of supernatural action is that it acts through the natural in
order to be truly supernatural.[15] This is true in both Christ's suffering
and filiation. On the one hand, human suffering in a divine mode is
a supernatural action. Indeed, Christ's limitless divine love is manifested in the world through the limited human action of suffering.[16] On the other hand, divine filiation in a human mode is also a
supernatural action. Christ's fully human life is the complete working out of his divine filiation.[17] For Williams, the infinite filial relation
between Father and Son, manifested in Christ's human suffering
and finitude, is the ground for all finite existence, including our own
filiation and suffering.[18]

Williams' Christology is indebted to the christological metaphysics of Maximus the Confessor. Andrew Louth calls Maximus'
christological vision a "Chalcedonian logic" that draws on the first
four ecumenical councils as a guide to the fundamental nature of
reality.[19] Maximus specifically uses the four adverbs from the Chalcedonian definition (without confusion, without change, without
division, without separation) as axiomatic for his understanding
of the integrity of created nature and its paradoxically necessary

relation with the divine for its fulfillment without blurring the Creator–creature distinction.

Applying Chalcedonian logic to Christ's divine–human person-hood who is "perfectly creaturely," we find the grounding for the metaphysical reality of the incarnation for understanding suffering and filiation in our own finite, human existence through a divine mode of existing. In the incarnation, human nature and its natural passions are united to Christ's hypostasis. Our human will became "unnatural" due to the fall but through divine power became nat-urally good once again. For Maximus, a naturally good will entails obedience to God.[20] Following Chalcedonian logic, Christ does human things divinely and divine things humanly.[21] In this way, God the Word suffered by way of the hypostatic union.[22]

A helpful conceptual innovation that Maximus provides is the distinction between *logos* and *tropos*, which elucidates the differ-ence between a subsistent thing's essence and its mode of existing. This distinction is vital to help us understand how a human can have a divine mode of existing. Maximus lays out the distinction between the *logos* of nature and the *tropos* of existence as a funda-mental metaphysical law:

> Every innovation, generally speaking, takes place in relation to the mode (*tropos*) of whatever is being innovated, not in relation to its principle (*logos*) of nature, because when a principle (*logos*) is innovated it effectively results in the destruction of nature, since the nature in question no longer possesses inviolate the principle (*logos*) according to which it exists. When, however, the mode (*tropos*) is innovated—so that the principle (*logos*) of nature is preserved inviolate—it manifests a wondrous power, for it displays nature being acted on and acting outside the lim-its of its own laws.[23]

Logos is the essence, the whatness of existence, whereas *tropos* is the *logos'* mode of existing, the how of existing. The distinction between *logos* and *tropos* is roughly that between the invariable and the variable in the life of a subsistent thing. The distinction allows Maximus to explain why sin does not change the definition of human nature, and how human nature can be raised to a new level of agency without transgressing the fundamental structure of nature.[24] In the incarnation, Christ's hypostasis unites the principle of human nature with the divine mode of existence in a perichoretic fashion to generate a new mode of existence in Christ's human flesh.[25] Put simply, *tropos* is the actualized, variable, lived-out dimension of one's invariable *logos* of nature.

So what is the *logos* of human nature? It is important to note that *logos* is not conceptually equivalent to "nature," which tends to have a static sense. Rather, *logos* has a dynamic sense, "shaping the activity of finite substance in the direction of its full and final actualization" and "defining the way in which an historical or temporal nature consistently grows into its optimal and complete identity, an identity in which its natural mode of existing is realized as fully as it can be in this or that particular subsistent reality within the world."[26] The *logos* of human nature participates beginning and end in *the Logos*, but human *logos* can have a *tropos* that aligns with or deviates away from its *logos*. So for humanity to be fully itself, it must be not only in complete alignment with its own natural *logos* but also in proper relationship with *the Logos*. If divine filiation is the proper mode of existing (*tropos*) for God the Word (*Logos*), and human *logos* is fulfilled in proper relationship with the *Logos*, then human *logos* is fulfilled in divine filiation as the divine mode of existing.[27] Maximus states explicitly that the purpose of the incarnation is deification of humanity that entails divine filiation: "The Word of God and God the Son of the Father became son of man and man himself for this reason, to make men gods and sons of God."[28] So the *logos* of human nature is paradoxically to transcend its nature and to be deified unto divine filiation as a divine mode of existing.

Having established the *logos* and *tropos* distinction, let us explore how Maximus' doctrine of the two wills of Christ is paradigmatic in the suffering of Jesus in Gethsemane, which affects our salvation and enables filiation as a divine mode of existing. The key point is that Christ's human will aligns with the divine will out of filial love for the sake of deification. Christ has two wills and two energies in accord with two natures. Based on the Chalcedonian logic, difference and union of the wills are meant to preserve the *logos* and the economy of salvation, respectively.[29] Because death entered by the exercise of free will in the garden of Eden, death needed to be reversed by Christ's human free will, which occurred in the garden of

Gethsemane.[30] Gethsemane demonstrates the weakness of Christ's flesh (in accordance with human flesh) and the perfect concordance between the will of the Father and the human will. Christ's human will is not deliberative but wholly natural in accordance with the divine will as it has been fully deified by virtue of the hypostatic union.[31]

The two wills of Christ enable divine filiation as a divine mode of existing for human creatureliness. Jesus' suffering in Gethsemane liberates the human will to align with the will of the Father, for "although he was a son, he learned obedience through what he suffered" (Heb 5:8, ESV).[32] Christ came to deify human nature in the hypostatic union and to show that the *logos* of human nature includes a divine *tropos*, which entails obedience and filiation to the Father.[33] As part of the divine economy, obedience to the will of the Father deifies the human nature.

Because of the divine power from his divine nature, Christ's human nature that necessarily hungers, thirsts, and fears death was willfully transformed into a divine mode of existing by voluntarily willing to hunger, thirst, and fear death.[34] Christ in Gethsemane rid human nature of its tendency to shrink away from death by doing human things divinely, which is willing to face death head on, and doing divine things humanly, which is willing to suffer for our sake. Maximus explains:

> For it appears that the same as man, who is also God by nature, wills in accordance with the economy that the cup pass, and in this he typifies what is human . . . so that he might take away all shrinking from death from our nature, and steel and arouse it to a brave assault against it, I mean against death. And again it appears that as God, being also a human being in essence, he wills to fulfill the economy of the Father and work the salvation of us all. It made clear then that as man, being by nature God, he acts humanly, willingly accepting the experience of suffering for our sake. And it is again made clear that as God, who is human by nature, he acts divinely and naturally exhibits the evidence of his divinity.[35]

By a kind of "fearful resolve in the face of death,"[36] Christ faced death in a divine mode of existing. Thus, by choosing to suffer and die in obedience to the will of the Father and love for us, Christ enacted a new mode of existence.

Through a divine mode of existing, Jesus paradoxically was more fully human: "'And in a manner beyond man, He truly became man,' since He maintained the modes of existence (which are above nature), along with the principles of being (which are according to nature), united and unimpaired."[37] To be fully human entails a divine mode of existing by grace while remaining human by nature. Crucially, Christ's divine mode of existing entails suffering unto divine filiation. Jesus' kenotic learning as a son through suffering is a model for human deification. As George Berthold has suggested, "Suffering is the tropos of deification."[38] Christ's sufferings are what Maximus calls "wondrous sufferings"[39] because they inaugurate a new divine way to experience emotions such as pain or the fear of death by orienting desire and aversion unto divine filiation.[40]

Therefore, deification does not entail willing whatever one wants, as with the transhumanists, enabled through technological manipulation of one's body, brain, or environment in order to overcome suffering. Rather, a divine mode of existing entails freedom to will in alignment with divine filiation, enabled through suffering. Choosing to submit to suffering unto the Father is the very mode of divine freedom and liberation. True deification entails a filiated will[41] over an exalted will. If human suffering is integral to Christ's Sonship, how much more should our human suffering be to our own status as a child of God? This is most apparent in the *theologia crucis*, to which we turn next.

Deification and the Theology of the Cross

Transhumanist Declaration proposition 1 states: "We envision the possibility of broadening human potential by overcoming aging, cognitive shortcomings, [and] involuntary suffering."[42] Limited lifespans and limited intelligence both contribute to the limitations of the human condition that result in suffering because they are rooted in death and finitude. Through the exercise of power via technology, suffering and death can be overcome. In this section we will explore how Luther's *theologia crucis* critiques this transhumanist power ontology.

Jeffrey Bishop has argued that transhumanism presupposes a Nietzschean power ontology, such that human will-to-power seeks to grow in ever greater ability to control and master the material world, including our own bodies.[43] Such a thirst for power is exactly what the theology of the cross is meant to oppose. The theology of the cross has its roots in Pauline theology, which Luther contrasts with the theology of glory. Transhumanist optimism in power unto auto-deification by technology is a kind of theology of glory. It is opposed to the suffering theology of the cross that is unto deification by grace and fulfillment in filiation.

Luther's theology of the cross rejects humanity's attempts at self-deification. At the core of the theology of the cross is the revelation of God: God reveals himself *through* suffering and the cross, not through the glory of human works. In the theology of glory, suffering is an offense to be avoided through relics, indulgences, and so forth, whereas the theology of the cross speaks of the hidden and crucified God and embraces the suffering of the cross.[44] Suffering in the form of "punishments, crosses, and death" are the "most sacred relics which the Lord of this theology himself has consecrated and blessed." Luther calls these relics of suffering "treasures" of "grace and glory" that are given only to "the most elect of the children of God."[45] Sufferings are graces that manifest the Christian's divine filiation. Luther draws out the corollary that lifelong repentance is the life of the cross "until death and thereby to entrance into the kingdom."[46] In other words, the whole of the Christian life entails suffering until death. Sons and daughters of God manifest their divine mode of existing through the sufferings of the cross.

Luther also critiques the theology of glory in its trust of power in varying dimensions. The theology of glory trusts in humanity's own abilities to save itself, whereas the theology of the cross calls on humanity to despair in its inability before receiving God's grace.[47] As theologians of glory, transhumanists trust in their own hands to save themselves from the plight of suffering and death through technological means.

Furthermore, the theology of the cross critiques the theology of glory's trust in the power of reason alone. The opposition is clear: theologians of glory are self-reliant unto auto-deification through reason while theologians of the cross are dependent on faith and grace for knowing God.[48] As Luther puts it, the true theologian recognizes God in suffering and the cross,[49] but, because of humanity's misuse of the knowledge of God through works, God sought to bring knowledge of God through suffering, which ultimately critiques human pride. The hiddenness of God lies within his suffering, so the theologian of glory does not know God or Christ. Thus, for Luther, true theology and knowledge of God are found only in suffering and the cross.[50] But if God reveals himself precisely through suffering and the cross, then theologians of glory *cannot* know God, especially when those theologians are the *ersatz* gods themselves, as in the case of transhumanism. The opposition between glory and the cross frustrates human attempts at self-deification.

The theology of the cross also critiques power unto virtue, contrasting human good works with the filial imitation of Christ. In the same way that the theology of the cross always brings low human pride, human virtue is also brought down and transformed, replacing self-conjured wisdom of the world with the gratitude of God's grace, manifested through the sufferings of the cross. The life of repentance and gratitude is a new, reborn life that, paradoxically, entails the "feeling of death."[51] The substance and telos of human virtue is Christoformity. Human works are only pleasing because they imitate Christ and are made possible by the grace of Christ with a filial faith.[52]

While Luther's theology of the cross effectively lays low the transhumanist desire for power as a theology of glory, more development of the theology of the cross is needed. Since there is no explicit account of deification in Luther's theology-of-the-cross discourses,[53] and Luther's theology of the cross originates with Pauline theology, we can draw on the growing scholarship on theosis in Pauline theology to further develop Luther's theology of the cross with deification as a central theme. For Paul, God is cruciform, and our cruciformity is deification.[54] Michael Gorman contends that Philippians 2:6–11 is Paul's master story.[55] He persuasively argues that the traditional translation of Philippians 2:6 as "although being in the form of God, did not consider his equality with God as something to be exploited for his own advantage" can be modified to "because being in the form of God." Due to the transition from "although" to "because," the sense of Philippians 2 is that the form of God has the very identity of kenosis and cruciformity.[56] Thus, if Christ is truly human, and the form of God in Christ is kenotic and

cruciform, then true humanity is cruciformity. Cruciformity is theo-
formity, and kenosis is theosis.[57]

For Paul, theosis is Christosis.[58] Ben Blackwell develops this
notion from a close reading of Romans 8, 2 Corinthians 4, and Philippians 3. Based on Romans 8:17–18, both "suffering with" and "glorified with" Christ sit under the overarching umbrella of conformity
to the image of Christ, which takes on a filial dimension. Conformity
to Christ entails a fuller obedience to the Father as Christ did. In
this way, suffering and glory in divine filiation reproduce the image
of Christ.[59] In 2 Corinthians 4:7–12, Christosis occurs through suffering and trials, revealing the life of God in the bodies of suffering
Christians. The experience of the life of Jesus comes through trials
that are embodied through the death of Jesus. Thus, the Christian
life embodies Christ's cruciform life through death "in the somatic
context of suffering so that Christ's image, characterized by death
and resurrection, is formed in them."[60] Living out Christ's resurrection still entails suffering. In Philippians 3:10–11, Paul emphasizes
suffering in resurrection life. Paul here again uses the language of
conformity to describe the "christoform nature of believers' experience," but this passage is unique in that the conformity language
focuses specifically on the aspect of suffering.[61] Like Luther's theology of the cross that seeks only to preach Christ and him crucified,
Christosis entails living out Christ and him crucified in the flesh
through suffering.

Christosis is a hidden transfiguration. The transfiguration
and the centrality of the cross are prominent themes in Maximus. Transfiguration highlights the eternal filial relationship in the
context of incarnation. Paul Blowers comments: "The transfiguration, as a theophany, has the advantage, first, of having grounded
revelation in *theologia*, the relation of Father and Son, and second, of doing so precisely in the context of the Son's incarnation.
Theologia and *oikonomia* dramatically intersect in the transfiguration."[62] Thus, Christ's suffering is a transfiguration; the suffering
of Christ in the flesh (*oikonomia*) reveals the Sonship of the Father
(*theologia*). Within the divine economy, God works to transfigure
humanity unto Christoformity and cruciformity as the beginning
of the transfiguration of the cosmos[63] and as the basis of Christ's
kingdom, which is characterized by humility and meekness shown

by Christ as the perfect human.[64] The logic of the divine economy is the cross:

> The mystery of the Incarnation of the Word bears the power of all the hidden *logos* and figures of Scripture as well as the knowledge of visible and intelligible creatures. The one who knows the mystery of the cross and the tomb knows the *logoi* of these creatures. And the one who has been initiated into the ineffable power of the resurrection knows the purpose for which God originally made all things.[65]

To know the cross is to know the heart of all God's dealings with his creation. Maximus' theology of the cross seeks to know Christ and him crucified and then elevate it to a cosmic reality.

The theology of the cross of Luther, Paul, and Maximus embraces power-in-weakness and grace through suffering and death, manifesting cruciformity. "To become God" is Christosis unto divine filiation. Such power-in-weakness and deification by suffering directly critiques the power ontology of transhumanism. Power-in-weakness is a divine mode of existing.

Deification and the Body of Christ

Transhumanist Declaration proposition 6 highlights the importance of "respecting autonomy and individual rights,"[66] which assumes a Western liberalism that is grounded upon an individualistic anthropology. There are contrasting visions of deification: one vision overcomes suffering, while the other suffers with one another in compassion. In this final section we will explore the ways Augustine's *totus Christus* as shared suffering critiques transhumanist individualism. Whereas transhumanism imagines humanity is surpassed when every individual can act as they wish without limitation, deification through suffering unto divine filiation occurs for the body of Christ, manifesting the virtues of Christ the Head, whose corporate identity critiques transhumanist individualism.

Augustine's notion of the *totus Christus*, the whole Christ, ties together the themes of suffering and transfiguration into the likeness of Christ the Head. Augustine grounds the *totus Christus* concept on the texts of Paul, with 1 Corinthians 12:12–27 being central.[67] Using Pauline ecclesiology as one of the exegetical keys for interpreting the Psalms, Augustine interweaves the suffering of Christ and his body as the suffering of the whole Christ with the goal of the transfiguration of the body as dependent children of God.

The *totus Christus* is the whole Christ as Christ is head and church is body.[68] While Christ does not need the body for completion, he chooses to be complete and entire with the church as his body. For Augustine, the whole Christ is the fullness of the church, as the completeness of a "certain perfect man (Eph 4:13), the man in whom we are each of us members."[69] Members of the church are constitutive of the whole Christ. So unified are Christ the Head and the church as his body that Christ experiences what Christians experience through his body, and Christians experience what is Christ's as their Head.[70] Because of the mystical union, Christ continues in suffering and even dying in the church, while the members of Christ's body rise in him.

The *totus Christus* is especially manifest in shared suffering between Christ and the members of his body. Suffering is a kind of speaking, which is carried on in the flesh of the members of the church as Christ's body since Christ is now in heaven. Note how Augustine patches together multiple Pauline passages to develop the theme of Christ's suffering in the body:

> The apostle desires *to fill up what is lacking to the sufferings of Christ in my own flesh* (Col 1:24). He speaks of *what is lacking* not to his own sufferings but *to the sufferings of Christ*, yet he prays that he may fill up this deficit not in the flesh of Christ but *in my own flesh*. He says that Christ is still suffering; but Christ cannot suffer in his own flesh, now glorified in heaven. Christ therefore suffers in my flesh, as it still struggles on earth. This is exactly what the apostle is telling us: Christ suffers in my flesh. *Now I live my own life no longer; it is Christ who lives in me* (Gal 2:20). If Christ himself were not truly suffering in his members, his faithful disciples, Saul could not possibly have been persecuting on earth the Christ who was enthroned in heaven. The former persecutor explains the matter clearly in another passage: *As your body is a unit and has many members, and yet all the members of the body, many though they be, are one body, so too is Christ* (1 Cor 12:12). Note that he does not say, "That is how it is with Christ and his body," but, *So too is Christ*. All of it is simply Christ, and because

the whole is Christ, the head shouted from heaven, *Saul, Saul, why are you persecuting me?* (Acts 9:4).[71]

The former Saul persecuted Christ by persecuting his body. But then he became the apostle Paul whose own suffering in the flesh filled up Christ's suffering. When the church suffers, Christ suffers not in his own flesh but in ours.[72] In this way, all of the suffering of Christ and his body is simply Christ, the whole Christ, suffering as one.

As the whole Christ, Christ is still suffering and laboring here on earth through the church. While Christ the Head has gone ahead, Christ follows in his body, as described in Matthew 25.[73] Christ is to be found among the poor, the sick, the imprisoned. To do the work of compassion is to serve and to suffer with the suffering Christ. Christ goes ahead as the marginalized one but then follows as the one who compassionately suffers through the members of the church.

Through the mystical union of the *totus Christus*, the church is transfigured particularly through suffering. Christ transfigures us into himself, such that Christ and his body speak through one another: "But in fact he who deigned to assume the form of a slave, and within that form to clothe us with himself, he who did not disdain to take us up into himself, did not disdain either to *transfigure us into himself*, and to speak in our words, so that we in our turn might speak in his."[74] The oneness and transfiguration of the whole Christ manifests in speech. The suffering of the church is a mode of Christ himself speaking. Augustine develops the theme of Christ in Gethsemane, noting that Christ the Head transfigures the body into himself by suffering through his body:

> He came to drain the cup of suffering and give salvation, he came to undergo death and give life. Facing death, then, because of what he had from us, he was afraid, not in himself but in us. When he said that his soul was sorrowful to the point of death, we all unquestionably said it with him. Without him, we are nothing, but in him we too are Christ. Why? Because the whole Christ consists of Head and body.[75]

When Christ was in Gethsemane and sorrowful to the point of death, the body of Christ was already saying it with him. The whole Christ speaks as one. Augustine goes on to invoke Acts 9:4 concerning Christ's calling out to Saul and the church's persecution, explaining that persecution of the *totus Christus* transfigures the church into Christ: "*Why are you persecuting me?* . . . is tantamount to asking, 'Why attack my limbs?' The Head was crying out on behalf of the members, and *the Head was transfiguring the members into himself.*"[76] Christ transfigures us so that he owns our suffering.[77]

However, that Christ owns our suffering is not an occasion for a sense of invincibility. The transfigured church as the body of Christ is empowered through dependence on Christ, her head: "All of us together with our Head are Christ, and without our Head we are helpless. . . . He can do plenty, or rather everything, without us, but we can do nothing without him."[78] Absolute dependence on Christ is part and parcel with conformity to Christ, which is enfleshed cruciformity. The power that the transfigured corporate body wields is power-in-weakness.

The *totus Christus* entails a wholeness in two directions: vertically between Christ and the church, and horizontally between members of the body. "If one member suffers, all suffer together" (1 Cor 12:26, ESV). The transhumanist might call this suffering together as one whole Christ to be weakness, something that should be engineered out through technological bioenhancement of individual power unto autonomous self-sufficiency. But such a view has no room for compassion, for "suffering with." Rather, Christ knows the suffering of the church because they are his own suffering. When any member of the body suffers, the whole body suffers. Shared suffering is a means to transfiguration into Christ's cruciformity. Suffering together, bound in love, is a divine mode of existing.

Conclusion

I have attempted to confront the transhumanist assumption about suffering by turning it on its head. Rather than autodeification by technology in order to overcome the problem of suffering, deification by grace is fulfilled precisely through suffering unto divine filiation. We saw that Christ fulfilled his divine mode of existing as the Word of God through his human suffering, submitting his human will to the divine will. Submission of the will as divine mode of existing directly opposes the transhumanist exaltation of the will. We then saw how the theology of the cross critiques the transhumanist power ontology. True divine power, manifested in the humility and meekness of the cross, is a suffering power-in-weakness. We finally saw how the *totus Christus* critiques transhumanist individualism through the corporate body of Christ, as a compassionate suffering together. The members of the body have their common identity as the whole Christ. Through suffering, the body is transfigured into Christ the Head. In conclusion, suffering itself is transfigured. Through suffering, humans become more human and paradoxically more divine. Suffering, not technological bioenhancement, is the true way to human enhancement.

But if we are to take Maximus' vision seriously, we must attend to the central importance of spiritual practice—that is, the lived dimension of the theology of suffering as human enhancement. The theology is only true if it is practiced in the body and as the body of Christ. It is one thing to theorize about suffering as divine *tropos*; it is quite another to live through suffering unto divine filiation.

As a concluding unscientific postscript, Kierkegaard's conception of truth-is-subjectivity illumines the reality that truth must be worked out existentially for the individual Christian: "The *how* of the truth is precisely the truth."[79] Following Kierkegaard's distinction between objective truth and subjective truth, the *how* of truth is more important than the *what* of truth. For example, imagine a speculative theologian who abstractly speaks about the objective truth of suffering unto divine filiation (such as the bulk of this chapter). But she becomes untruth the moment she curses God when stricken with painful suffering of her own. Conversely, imagine a lay Christian who lacks theological sophistication and cannot make heads or tails of "suffering unto divine filiation." But when she is faced with painful suffering, she grows deeper in faith and dependence on God the Father, manifesting a divine mode of existing as divine filiation. This lay Christian embodies the truth in her subjectivity, whereas the speculative theologian lives untruth.[80] Indeed, the key is to "comprehend the secret of suffering as the form of the highest life."[81]

If what I have been arguing about suffering unto divine filiation is true, then Kierkegaardian truth-is-subjectivity provides helpful, practical implications. First, since the truth of suffering unto divine filiation must be worked out subjectively, one cannot view the spiritual efficacy of suffering as wholly effective in a mechanistic way.

Deification as effect does not come about simply by suffering as a kind of efficient cause. This conception falls into the trap of technologizing grace, such that suffering is viewed as a kind of technology that instrumentally guarantees a desired effect. Second, suffering ought not be used as a tool of abuse. One cannot abstractly lecture to a sufferer about suffering unto deification in the manner of Kierkegaardian objective truth. Rather, suffering for deification can be addressed only for oneself or through compassionate encounter with the sufferer—a suffering with—in the manner of subjective truth. If suffering unto deification is for divine filiation, then one cannot prescribe suffering for a spiritual brother or sister, but instead suffering must be entered into as collective members of the *totus Christus*. Finally, since there is a divine call to enter into the suffering of another, one cannot be opposed in principle to the relief of suffering through medical means. Use of medicine can be a manifestation of God's mercy, which is an occasion for growth in dependence on God and divine filiation.

While suffering is not an intrinsic good, suffering is a transfiguring means by which the intrinsic good of divine filiation makes us fully human in a divine mode of existing. Transhumanist auto-deification that exalts will, power, and individual self appears impotent and impoverished in the face of such a powerful vision of divine, familial love.

NOTES

1   Max More, "The Philosophy of Transhumanism," in *The Transhumanist Reader*, ed. Max More and Natasha Vita-More (Malden, Mass.; Oxford: Wiley-Blackwell, 2013), 4.

2   "Transhumanist FAQ Live," entry in *H+Pedia*, accessed December 8, 2021, https://hpluspedia.org/wiki/Transhumanist_FAQ_Live.

3   More, "Philosophy of Transhumanism," in More and Vita-More, *Transhumanist Reader*, 4.

4   Nick Bostrom, "Human Genetic Enhancements: A Transhumanist Perspective," *Journal of Value Inquiry* 37, no. 4 (2003): 493–506.

5   More, "Philosophy of Transhumanism," in More and Vita-More, *Transhumanist Reader*, 14.

6   Ingmar Persson and Julian Savulescu, *Unfit for the Future: The Need for Moral Enhancement* (New York: Oxford University Press, 2012).

7   Ronald Cole-Turner, "Going Beyond the Human: Christians and Other Transhumanists," *Theology and Science* 13, no. 2 (2015): 150–61.

8   King-Ho Leung, "The Technologisation of Grace and Theology: Metatheological Insights from Transhumanism," *Studies in Christian Ethics* 33, no. 4 (2020): 479–95.

9   For example, see Eugenia Torrance, "Acquiring Incorruption: Maximian Theosis and Scientific Transhumanism," *Studies in Christian Ethics* 32, no. 2 (2019): 177–86; Simeon Zahl, "Engineering Desire: Biotechnological Enhancement as Theological Problem," *Studies in Christian Ethics* 32, no. 2 (2019): 216–28; Brandon Gallaher, "Godmanhood vs Mangodhood: An Eastern Orthodox Response to Transhumanism," *Studies in Christian Ethics* 32, no. 2 (2019): 200–215.

10   By "filiation," I mean the condition of being a child of God. "Filiation" is used instead of "adoption" because the former encompasses both the eternal Sonship of the second person of the Trinity and the adoptive child status of humans. Human adoptive filiation is fulfilled in imaging the divine filiation of Christ through deification.

11   It is acknowledged that both a coherent philosophy of technology and a taxonomy of different kinds of suffering are necessary to help discern which technologies are permissible in relieving suffering, but they are beyond the scope of this chapter.

12   "Transhumanist Declaration," entry in *H+Pedia*, last revised 2009, accessed December 8, 2021, https://hpluspedia.org/wiki/Transhumanist_Declaration.

13   Rowan Williams, *Christ the Heart of Creation* (London: Bloomsbury, 2018), xiii.

14   Williams, *Christ*, 226.

15   Williams, *Christ*, 4.

16   Williams, *Christ*, 21.

17   Williams, *Christ*, 32.

18   Williams, *Christ*, 242.

19   Andrew Louth, introduction to *Maximus the Confessor*, by Maximus the Confessor, trans. Andrew Louth, The Early Church Fathers (New York: Routledge, 1996), 22–23.

20   Maximus the Confessor, *Ambiguum* 4, PG 91.1041D–1044A. For an English translation, see Maximos the Confessor, *On Difficulties in the Church Fathers: The Ambigua*, trans. Nicholas Constas, 2 vols. (Cambridge, Mass.: Harvard University Press, 2014).

21   Maximus, *Ambiguum* 5, PG 91.1044CD (trans. Constas, 1:27–29).

22   Maximus, *Ambiguum* 5, PG 91.1044D–1045A.

23   Maximus, *Ambiguum* 42, PG 91.1341D (trans. Constas, 2:173).

24   Williams, *Christ*, 101.

25   Maximus, *Ambiguum* 5, PG 91.1053B–C (trans. Constas, 1:45).

26   Williams, *Christ*, 102–3.

27   Williams, *Christ*, 105, 108.

28   Maximus the Confessor, *Capita theologica et oeconomica* II.25. For an English translation, see Maximus the Confessor, *Maximus Confessor: Selected Writings*, trans. George C. Berthold, Classics of Western Spirituality (New York: Paulist, 1985), 152–53.

29   Maximus the Confessor, *Opusculum* 7, PG 91.84A–B. For an English translation, see Maximus the Confessor, *Maximus the Confessor* (trans. Andrew Louth).

30   Maximus, *Ambiguum* 7, PG 91.1076AB.

31   Maximus, *Opusculum* 7, PG 91.80CD, 81C–84A. Maximus famously makes a distinction between the natural will and the gnomic will, arguing that Christ has two natural wills but not two gnomic wills. The natural will is akin to the capacity or disposition to will according to nature, whereas gnomic will is akin to actualization or exercising of willing. Put differently, natural will is defined by nature, while gnomic will is defined by person. If Christ had two gnomic wills, then Christ would be schizophrenic with an internal battle between active wills. But since Christ has two natural wills, Christ's human will is always disposed to will in alignment with its proper human nature and cannot deliberate contrary to its nature, for contrary to human nature would be in opposition to God. Only human gnomic will, not natural will, can be opposed to God. In light of the following discussion, we will see that, for Maximus, Christ fears death as a part of the natural will, and he can even be tempted (Heb 4:15), but he cannot be inclined to sin due to lack of gnomic will. See Maximus the Confessor, *Opusculum* 3, PG 91.45B–48C, 56AB.

32   Paul M. Blowers, *Maximus the Confessor: Jesus Christ and the Transfiguration of the World* (Oxford: Oxford University Press, 2016), 234.

33   Maximus, *Opusculum* 7, PG 91.77B–80B (trans. Louth, 184–85).

34   Maximus, *Ambiguum* 5, PG 91.1053C.

35   Maximus, *Opusculum* 7, PG 91.84BC (trans. Louth, 188).

36   Blowers, *Maximus*, 238.

37   Maximus, *Ambiguum* 5, PG 91.1056A (trans. Constas, 1:49).

38   Maximus, *Maximus Confessor*, 173, n. 57.

39   Maximus, *Ambiguum* 5, PG 91.1056AB.

40   Blowers, *Maximus*, 239.

41 By "filiated will," I mean a will that is defined by its obedience to the Father in accordance with being a child of God.

42 "Transhumanist Declaration," entry in *H+Pedia*, last revised 2009, accessed December 8, 2021, https://hpluspedia.org/wiki/Transhumanist_Declaration.

43 Jeffrey P. Bishop, "Nietzsche's Power Ontology and Transhumanism: Or Why Christians Cannot Be Transhumanists," in *Christian Perspectives on Transhumanism and the Church: Chips in the Brain, Immortality, and the World of Tomorrow*, ed. Steve Donaldson and Ron Cole-Turner (Cham, Switzerland: Palgrave Macmillan, 2018), 117–35.

44 Ronald K. Rittgers, *The Reformation of Suffering: Pastoral Theology and Lay Piety in Late Medieval and Early Modern Germany* (Oxford: Oxford University Press, 2012), 112.

45 Martin Luther, "Explanations of the Ninety-Five Theses," trans. Carl W. Folkemer, in *Luther's Works, Volume 31: Career of the Reformer I*, ed. Harold J. Grimm (Philadelphia: Fortress, 1957), 225–26.

46 Luther, "Explanations," 89.

47 Martin Luther, "Heidelberg Disputation, 1518," trans. Harold J. Grimm, in Grimm, *Luther's Works, Volume 31*, 40.

48 Rittgers, *Reformation*, 112.

49 Luther, "Heidelberg Disputation," 40.

50 Luther, "Heidelberg Disputation," 53.

51 Luther, "Heidelberg Disputation," 55.

52 Luther, "Heidelberg Disputation," 56–57.

53 The "Finnish School" of Luther interpretation claims that Luther's doctrine of justification by faith entails a doctrine of *theosis*, arguing that the latter corresponds to effective justification with Christ ontically present in faith. For Tuomo Mannermaa, the founder of the Finnish School, "the goal of the *theologia crucis* is precisely *theosis*." Mannermaa, "Justification and *Theosis* in Lutheran-Orthodox Perspective," in *Union with Christ: The New Finnish Interpretation of Luther*, ed. Carl E. Braaten and Robert W. Jenson (Grand Rapids: Eerdmans, 1998), 39.

54 Michael J. Gorman, *Inhabiting the Cruciform God: Kenosis, Justification, and Theosis in Paul's Narrative Soteriology* (Grand Rapids: Eerdmans, 2009), 1–2.

55 Gorman, *Inhabiting*, 12–13.

56 Gorman, *Inhabiting*, 24–25.

57 Gorman, *Inhabiting*, 37.

58 Ben C. Blackwell, *Christosis: Engaging Paul's Soteriology with His Patristic Interpreters*, rev. ed. (Grand Rapids: Eerdmans, 2016).

59 Blackwell, *Christosis*, 162–63, 167.

60 Blackwell, *Christosis*, 203.

61 Blackwell, *Christosis*, 206–7.

62 Blowers, *Maximus*, 79.

63 Blowers, *Maximus*, 134.

64 Maximus, *Ambiguum* 32, PG 91.1284CD.

65 Maximus, *Capita theologica et oeconomica* I.66 (trans. Berthold, 139–40). Translation slightly modified.

66 "Transhumanist Declaration," entry in *H+Pedia*, last revised 2009, accessed December 8, 2021, https://hpluspedia.org/wiki/Transhumanist_Declaration.

67 Tarsicius J. van Bavel, "The 'Christus Totus' Idea: A Forgotten Aspect of Augustine's Spirituality," in *Studies in Patristic Christology*, ed. Thomas Finan and Vincent Twomey (Dublin: Four Courts Press, 1998), 84–85.

68 Augustine, *Sermon 341*, in *Sermons 341–400: The Works of Saint Augustine III/10*, trans. Edmund Hill (Hyde Park, N.Y.: New City Press, 1995), 26.

69 Augustine, *Sermon 341*, 19.

70 Augustine, *Exposition of Psalm 100*, §3, in *Expositions of the Psalms 99–120: The Works of Saint Augustine III/19*, trans. Maria Boulding (Hyde Park, N.Y.: New City Press, 2004), 33.

71 Augustine, *Exposition of Psalm 142*, §3, in *Expositions of the Psalms 121–150: The Works of Saint Augustine III/20*, trans. Maria Boulding (Hyde Park, N.Y.: New City Press, 2004), 346 (emphasis original).

72 Bavel, "Christus Totus," in Finan and Twomey, *Studies*, 89.

73 Augustine, *Exposition of Psalm 86*, §5, in *Expositions of the Psalms 73–98: The Works of Saint Augustine III/18*, trans. Maria Boulding (Hyde Park, N.Y.: New City Press, 2002), 251.

74 Augustine, *Second Exposition of Psalm 30*, §3, in *Expositions of the Psalms 1–32: The Works of Saint Augustine III/15*, trans. Maria Boulding (Hyde Park, N.Y.: New City Press, 2000), 322–23 (emphasis added).

75 Augustine, *Second Exposition of Psalm 30*, §3, 323.

76 Augustine, *Second Exposition of Psalm 30*, §3, 323 (emphasis added).

77 J. David Moser, "Corpus Mysticum: A Response to Vanhoozer, Horton, and Allen," *Pro Ecclesia* 29, no. 1 (2020): 64.

78 Augustine, *Second Exposition of Psalm 30*, §4, 324–25.

79 Søren Kierkegaard, *Concluding Unscientific Postscript to Philosophical Fragments*, ed. Howard V. Hong and Edna H. Hong (Princeton, N.J.: Princeton University Press, 1992), 1:323 (emphasis original).

80 Kierkegaard, *Concluding*, 1:202–3.

81 Kierkegaard, *Concluding*, 1:444.

6
THIS IS MY BODY

Faith Communities as Sites of Transfiguring Vulnerability

Wylin D. Wilson

There was palpable electricity in the air as I entered the unadorned sanctuary full of bodies that were alive with nervous, hopeful, and fearful energy. The bodies in this modest church building, just off a rural Alabama highway, were not like the ones in typical middle- and upper-middle-class church congregations. These bodies were visibly uncomfortable, shaken: some of them disheveled and bent over; others seemed ashamed (maybe because their clothes were unwashed and smelled of a mixture of dirt and alcohol). Others were rocking, not to music, but to a personal cadence accompanied by a dazed facial expression and quiet murmuring. I found this congregation full of different bodies refreshing. There was constant movement and freedom that came with the welcoming embrace of members who made it clear that somatic, cognitive, and demographic difference was the norm in this place. Some of the individuals were reentering society from the carceral system and recovering from substance abuse; others were homeless and uncomfortable being in spaces that were usually associated with being unwelcoming to those who did not dress or look like "respectable, sober Christians." The services in this church were never predictable, always exciting, and sometimes noisy—unlike what most people expect when attending church services where the ushers, members, and leadership make it clear that quiet and conformity are expected.

This small rural church is a site of transfiguring vulnerability. Because people become vulnerable through social norms and practices that ensnare individuals in relationships of hierarchy and unjust economic and political structures,[1] vulnerability often indicates existence on the margins within societal and ecclesial spaces. In addition to the common perception of the margins as spaces for those who are excluded and devalued, the margins are also "lively space[s] of creative energy, place[s] of Spirit."[2] The Spirit is "a power that connects members of the community, [catalyzes] healing by empowering creative agency, not simply by including the helpless or by restoring somatic intactness, but opening a physical social space of non-domination and mutuality."[3] Where this Spirit is, there is freedom from the critical theological and cultural gazes that diminish the value of those who are different and perceived as limited. Therefore, transfiguring vulnerability happens when congregations, through prophetic witness, genuine and deep access, nurture a communion of vulnerable and caring mutuality[4] without barriers "that is created by all and for all, in which people with disabilities [and with various ethnic, racial, class, sexual orientation, and gender differences] are valued among others as contributing members."[5] Transfiguring vulnerability happens when, instead of demanding that others come to them, churches move to the lively spaces of creative energy and places of Spirit—the margins, where difference and grace abound. When Christ beckons individuals to come to him, the call accompanies Christ's movement toward others, not a command of a recalcitrant Savior unwilling to move to the creative space of Spirit where difference is embodied and embraced.

Ultimately, transfiguring vulnerability is the act of reinterpreting limits and cultivating practices of deep accessibility, robust hospitality, attentiveness, and solidarity, aiming for the eschatological hope of radical acceptance and full inclusion of difference within a congregation. The transfiguring power of Christ's call to come is what animates the biblical prophetic witness of the church. The original Greek for "transfigure" means "supernaturally transformed." Examining the biblical narrative of Christ's transfiguration is useful in helping us further grasp practical ways that congregations can become sites of transfiguring vulnerability.

This chapter begins by illustrating transfiguring vulnerability, and a discussion of how transhumanists and Christians understand it differently ensues. At the heart of these divergent understandings is the problem that embodiment poses for transhumanists and Christians. Examining bioenhancement as an outcome of perceiving body as "frontier" buttresses this discussion of embodiment. The chapter ends by demonstrating how churches can transfigure vulnerability through practices of deep accessibility, robust hospitality, attentiveness, and solidarity, all of which build on the foundation of a reinterpretation of limits and an eschatological approach to the problem of the body in Christianity.

TRANSFIGURATION

The account of the transfiguration in the Gospel of Mark (Mark 9:2–9) records the events on a high mountain ascended by Jesus and three of his disciples: Peter, James, and John. On the mountain, Christ is transfigured (symbolized by his inimitably luminous clothing) before them, and Elijah and Moses appear and talk with Jesus. Culminating this display of Christ's glory is a cloud that overshadows them and the audible voice of God affirming Christ's identity as God's Beloved Son. This narrative, which is recorded within all synoptic gospels, is significant because of its rich symbolism and association with Jewish apocalyptic tradition. Complexity shrouds the interpretation of this story, as some scholars argue that it is a misplaced story of Christ's resurrection, while others highlight its eschatological and apocalyptic significance.[6]

Jewish and Christian apocalyptic literature is commonly characterized by eschatological imagery and meaning; however, biblical scholars also note that apocalyptic literature is not limited to eschatological narratives, but they also focus on "the direct revelation of heavenly mysteries . . . that certain individuals are given to understand the mysteries of God, man [sic] and the universe."[7] Noteworthy is Christ's glorification, displayed by his clothing, which is illustrative of the exalted state of a heavenly being or holy person.[8] Within the Old Testament, God's glory is predominantly portrayed as shining brilliance or bright light.[9] Jesus' divinity is further confirmed when Peter suggests that they make "tents" or "Tabernacles," which are places of habitation for divine beings or righteous ones within Jewish tradition. Furthermore, the appearance of Elijah and Moses signify the establishment of God's kingdom: "Moses appears as the representative of the old covenant and the promise, now shortly to be fulfilled in the death of Jesus, and Elijah as the appointed restorer of all things. . . . The stress on Elijah's presence at the transfiguration indicates that the fulfilment of 'all things' has arrived."[10] Likewise, the divine proclamation upon their being enveloped by the cloud, which was a repetition of God's affirmation of Christ's unique identity as God's Son during his baptism, also reveals Christ's glory—which seemed so often hidden in his daily experience with the disciples that they often displayed ignorance of Christ's full character and true identity as God incarnate:

> The transfiguration . . . has disclosed a new aspect of God's truth: Jesus himself the new Tabernacle of divine glory. His word and deed transcend all past revelation. This was the truth with which the disciples were confronted when they realized they were once again alone in the presence of Jesus.[11]

Just as the cloud and change in Christ's raiment revealed the often veiled fullness of who he was as the Son of God, we often do not recognize the fullness of who others are in our midst. Often, this world does not see others as bearers of the Holy Spirit, whole, loved, and worthy of equal regard. Instead, when people encounter difference in others, they often see them as limited, unworthy, in need of enhancement to fit ideals that mark loveable, worthy bodies. Theology and ecclesial spaces are also culpable in perpetuating detrimental stigmatizing narratives regarding differently "marked" bodies (marked by ability, race, class, gender, sexual orientation, and ethnicity). However, various theologians have displayed the moral courage to proclaim a God not only who lives among us but also whose marks mirror our own in significant ways—ways that stand courageously against societal violence against such marked bodies.[12]

Through mass media, cultural symbols, and norms, modern individuals receive the mediated message that "almost every body is 'failed' in some respect."[13] There is often dissatisfaction with the somatic individual, because it does not meet some imposed "norm" with respect to culturally mediated values of ability, health, or aesthetic measure. In the quest for a "true self," liberty, perfection, and normalization,[14] "technologies for . . . transforming the body proliferate, organizing themselves around ever more fine-grained and idealized norms of beauty and self-management."[15] Bioenhancement, reflecting the cultural obsession with bodily perfection, is one significant consequence of conceptualizing the body as "frontier." The cultural touchstone of the "frontier" conjures images of space that is not fully explored or is undeveloped. Just as scientific and technological advancements allow us to imagine the possibility of settling frontiers such as outer space or the deep sea, biomedical innovations along with advances in computer and information science, engineering, and nanotechnology allow us to explore and imagine manipulating and conquering the body in ways previously thought impossible.

The uncritical acceptance of body as "frontier" has coincided with transhumanism's perception of the body as a site of scientific and technological conquest—a frontier to be seized in the battle against human limits. Moreover, when our cultural renderings of optimism and progress combine with envisioning phenomena as frontier, it can create precarious consequences. For these cultural renderings of optimism and progress, among other things, shape the American moral imagination. Thus, the narratives that influence our imaginings about our perceived linear course toward a "better" or utopian future are born of historical visions that do not delineate harmful connections between notions of progress, optimism, and exceptionalism. Our historical narrative of progress and exceptionalism does not take into account the underside of our progress, which comes at the cost of marginalized human lives and our ecological well-being. Acknowledgment of an expansive view of history recognizes that the "uncritical celebration of the 'frontier' as a site of boundless freedom and creativity . . . has had disastrous consequences for America's internal and external others."[16] Moreover, this notion of a limitless frontier to be occupied and conquered not only has serious implications for the environment upon which life depends but, regarding the body, has led to questions about human nature—what makes us human, and how far we can go with bioenhancement before we are no longer human (i.e., posthuman).

Furthermore, the perceived necessity of bioenhancement is partly ingrained in the historical denigration of marginalized bodies, stemming from the erroneous association between moral character and bodies marked by difference.[17] Bodies that fall outside of society's definition of what is normative are often vilified and deemed unworthy of protection and honor. However, vulnerable bodies that are held up to the critical cultural gaze of normalization and found lacking can be embraced by faith communities practicing radical hospitality. These faith communities can create places where, even if society sees incompleteness and unsoundness, their embrace can be a needed source of healing for bodies suffering discrimination, exclusion, and violence.

The Christian church, as an expression of Christ's body, is a site where practical ways of transfiguring vulnerability can manifest. This chapter examines how faith communities—through the practical work of embodying Christ, prophetic witness, and activism—can help humanity understand the insidious effects of normalization. The danger of normalization is that the identity of vulnerable bodies and selves is defined by their relationship to culturally imposed norms that can lead to othering, excluding, and, in its most insidious form, inciting violence against those who do not "measure up." Faith communities can offer not just prophetic witness and activism against such exclusion and violence but practical ways of being more humane. Embodying Christ is fundamental to envisioning how transfiguring vulnerability plays out practically within faith communities. Christ's physical and symbolic body (the church) are both sites of power and vulnerability. Before we explore more details of practical ways that transfiguring vulnerability is displayed through Christ's contemporary body of the church, we will examine a foundational issue for this chapter: the relationship between embodiment and transhumanism.

The Problem of Embodiment and Transhumanism

Our scientific and technological innovations are so much a part of the modern somatic individual—we ingest, play, and wear them. From pharmacological and cognitive inventions to artificial intelligence, humanity has been transformed through science and technology. The possibilities created by and the pace at which innovations occur within science and technology fuel an expansive imaginary of who and what humanity can do and become. Movements such as transhumanism laud what science and technology can make possible for human flourishing. Generally, proponents of transhumanism extol the transformative powers of science and technology for their ability to subdue suffering, surmount death, and defeat disease. This "techno–utopian" (or extropian) framework maintains that technology and science can not only improve the human condition but move humans beyond current limitations, into a posthuman form. There is much diversity within this intellectual movement, from those who eschew religion to Christian transhumanists who understand Christianity to affirm humans as scientific and technological creatures.[18]

The ideal at the center of transhumanism is a hyper–autonomous, unencumbered, unembedded, and disembodied individual. This individual has morphological freedom and is conceptualized devoid of *relational* autonomy, which considers deep embeddedness within communities and relationships that have moral claims on individuals. Indeed, transhumanists seek escape not only from the limitations of embodiment but from all troubling aspects of materiality. Thus, some seek human enhancements that allow humanity to survive life beyond "narrow environmental conditions,"[19] and others seek escape from Earth.[20] Christian theologian Norman Wirzba correctly responds to this "transhumanist urge" to escape materiality. He contends that instead of seeking to escape this world through virtual or interstellar means, we should focus on transforming the desires and habits that not only render our world uninhabitable but render human relationships inhospitable.[21] The significance of the transfiguration of vulnerability is the practical illustration of Wirzba's concern. The focus of transhumanism is on the somatic individual—getting the body right, whereas the focus of the Christian notion of transfiguring vulnerability is getting right with Others—people, God, and creation. Therefore, the concern is respecting relational autonomy and being in right relationship with Others.

Bioenhancement is central to human flourishing and continued existence for transhumanists. For instance, Natasha Vita–More, one of the leading proponents and first female philosophers of the movement, views aging not as a natural process but as a disease state and claims that human enhancement is a matter of survival.[22] Beginning as a fringe intellectual phenomenon, transhumanism has grown into a global social movement, garnering the support of individuals seeking to push political action and policies that proponents believe will facilitate morphological freedom and surpass the limits of human nature through science and technology. Within

Europe and the United States, transhumanism has evolved into a social movement that has evident roots within Enlightenment humanism, and there are proponents in various countries who work to mobilize political support for human enhancement advocacy.[23] The possibilities unfolding from the transhumanist imaginary revive age-old questions regarding anthropology, ontology, and soteriology. Technological innovations and scientific advancements have precipitated reconsiderations of human nature and limits. Ron Cole-Turner purports:

> We are former human beings who no longer remember what we once were but cannot imagine what we will soon become. Where will it all come out? I haven't a clue. But I am certain that we will be different from what we were in the past and what we are even now. We live suspended between old and new, on a zip line between the familiar and the unimaginable. . . . Welcome to the world of "trans-." We are all transforming or transitioning from one thing to another. We are reinventing ourselves without a blueprint or a goal. For some, human reinvention is scary. For others, it is liberating and exciting. For most of us, it brings mixed feelings.[24]

Cole-Turner captures the continuum of perspectives regarding human enhancement from ambivalence to exuberance. He implies that transhumanism holds out the promise that we can be something more than (i.e., better than) human. Inherent in its prospect of reinvention is the luring notion that transhumanism seems to allow individuals to transcend religion's circumscription of imperfect human experience and fate. Transhumanism seems to offer the elimination of the uncertainty that comes with religious beliefs regarding salvation and death. It seems to be an effort to wrest humanity's fate from the hands of God and offer a brand of liberation from the somatic limitations that burden humanity with biological, cognitive, and emotional shackles. Therefore, instead of being static, human nature is a "work-in-progress, a half-baked beginning that we can learn to remold in desirable ways."[25] Transhumanism, however, does not stand alone in its struggle with embodiment.

EMBODIMENT: ALSO A CHRISTIAN STRUGGLE

Scholars have tried to navigate the problematic nature of the body within the history of philosophy, science, and religion. Within

Christianity, the body is a theological problem,[26] as it is both affirmed as good through God's proclamation of delight in creation and understood as originator of unruly passions and sinful desires after the fall. For many Christians, bodies need to be under the authority of an outside spiritual or political governing force—particularly, those bodies that fall outside social "norms." In a similar vein, transhumanism's reduction of the body to a mere site of domination and manipulation for the sake of human happiness is a precarious path to the reduction of bodies to objects. As objects, bodies can be used as clinical material (for experimentation) and "frontiers" to be developed. Transhumanism is one approach to the problem of embodiment; however, the Christian theologian Scott MacDougall presents an eschatological approach to the problem of the body in Christianity. He posits:

> In the eschatological light of Christ's resurrection, the body appears not as a temporary and disposable flesh envelope for a "soul" or "spirit" enclosed within it, a non-material essence that is the "real" person, but the concrete and highly complex formation of a unique identity produced by the confluence of biological materiality, social and cultural processes, and transpersonal relational narratives. The body . . . is an infinitely beloved creature of God that does not lose its creatureliness or escape its finitude, but that, resurrected—somehow—as "spiritual body" in the Pauline sense, is able to inhabit the perfected creation of God's eschatological promise (depicted scripturally as the new heaven and new earth) with a freedom in relation to time and space that bodies now do not possess.[27]

Within such an eschatological framework, "the body is the locus of personal identity"; thus, individuals do not *have* a body but *are* their bodies.[28] Therefore, the transhumanist reduction of the body to a mere material "substrate" is untenable within Christianity. Although science and technological advances have shifted the imaginary of humans regarding suffering, death, and salvation, transhumanism's claims regarding the possibility of mastering human weakness and limitation may be particularly unsatisfying for individuals embedded in communities of care. In the face of suffering and death, Christian communities that embody Christlike love and sacrifice through compassionate care can help ease the psychological disturbance caused by human vulnerability.

Embodiment is marked by vulnerability and dependency; however, Christ's own marked embodiment through the incarnation is an affirmation that our limited bodies are good. At the same time, the diversity of human embodiment renders some bodies more vulnerable than others. It is here that we must remember that the body of Christ, as church, includes diversity. Therefore, social identity markers such as race, class, gender, ability, and ethnicity ought not be seen as deficient, as doing so puts these bodies at risk. The body of Christ, marked by identities contrary to normative power and authority in his lifetime, was wounded and raised in humiliation on the cross, but he stood as a testimony to the miracle of God's ability to restore wholeness in a world that denies dignity to those deemed unworthy and unfit.

From the beginning, the human body of the Divine Self in Christ was problematic.[29] Christ was born into cultural and religious subjugation because of his particular embodiment. Likewise, the continued embodiment of Christ through the church has historically stood confounded by cultural practices, prohibitions, and self-understandings that have left individuals confused about just what it means to *be* the continued presence of Christ's body in the world.

Throughout history, Christians have clumsily navigated theological and practical notions of embodiment. The church in European and American history is implicated in the brutalization and disregard for various bodies marked by difference.[30] The church has been used as an instrument of upholding economic and political control by providing the ideological scaffolds that sanction pilfering and subjugation of indigenous and other racialized and gendered marginalized bodies. Furthermore, bodies that fall short of the cultural "norms" are often held within disapproving societal gazes that limit how their worth is perceived by society. However, audacious scholarship of feminist, black, LGBTQ+, and disability theologians who dare to claim that God dwells among us in bodies that are marked like ours is leading congregations in subversive, transfiguring work. These congregations' basis for love and care of non-normative flesh is an incarnate God who intimately identifies with us—especially in our varied embodiment.[31]

The first churches found themselves in a similar predicament. The first-century church was instrumental in the moral formation of Christians who were religious minorities within Greco-Roman society. The church had a critical posture toward Jewish religious authorities who upheld religious rites, laws, and social hierarchy. "Jesus and early Christianity transformed standard cultural patterns of moral relationships, making them less hierarchical and status-oriented and more inclusive and compassionate."[32] Lisa Cahill attests to the difficult task of modern Christians to continue cultivating and creating moral practices and ways of being that "enable the church to have the same transformative cultural effect it had in the first century—however incipiently, incompletely, and sometimes retrogressively."[33] In light of the "transhumanist urge," the biblical narrative of the transfiguration yields insight into how contemporary Christians can continue the generative work of the church that enables individuals to cope with dissatisfaction with embodied existence and preoccupation with sustaining health and well-being amid suffering, addiction, illness, and death.

Transfiguring Vulnerability through Reinterpretation

Philosophies like transhumanism subject individuals to the "tyranny of the normal"[34]—in this view, bodies need enhancements because they do not measure up to norms of function, skill, and aesthetics. There are dominating ideals that continue to shape who and what attributes are valued. An important question that we must ask ourselves is, what would be the task of transhumanism if we *valued* human limits and disability? Furthermore, what would be its task if "the recognition of limits [was] . . . not . . . tied uncritically to interpretations of value and worth"?[35] Deborah B. Creamer offers an imaginary that is significant as we try to answer these questions, particularly for congregations seeking to transfigure vulnerability. She offers a model for communal practice and theological reflection that reinterprets limits and disability.[36] For Creamer, disability does not belong solely to the realm of care, and human limits are valued. In her reinterpretation, limits are not a deficit but "lead us toward creativity, even toward God."[37] This reinterpretation is at the root of what it means for congregations to transfigure vulnerability.

The commonly used notion of *limited*—which signifies deficiency and incapability, and emphasizes impediments and constraints—is replaced by a conception of *limits* as a "normal and unsurprising aspect of life"[38] that indicates a "quality of being—one *has* limits."[39] Creamer argues that when our beginning assumption is able-bodied normality, we think of disability as "limited"—what is not normal. Furthermore, within a medical model, disability represents lack, something that needs to be fixed. However, within a limits model, disability is not repugnant or aberrant but what commonly marks our embodied selves. Although our limits are stigmatized, Creamer helps transform limits from being demonized into being good, normalized. This normalization shifts the position of "disability and difference from the margins as an exceptional and othering experience."[40]

Indeed, transhumanists' refusal to accept the limits of embodiment, such as aging and death, is a form of denial that has the potential to harm "those on whom we project and reject these limits, the environment (when we pretend that it also has no limits), and even ourselves."[41] In her advocacy of theological reflection and practices of "messy, complicated embodiment, including the prevalence of limits,"[42] Creamer is not implying that we should not seek to surmount or adapt to limits. She would not suggest that we abandon human enhancements. Likewise, we should not have a wholesale acceptance of all limits. Some harmful limits should be spurned—violence and poverty, for instance.[43] Creamer's limits model facilitates the rejection of labels, makes our assumptions and barriers more clear, and provides us with a more authentic conceptualization of embodiment in its full complexity.[44] Thus, adapting Creamer's paradigm within our theological reflection and actual practice has the potential to transform how we understand others and ourselves as well as how we relate to one another.

Disability theologian Thomas Reynolds offers a template for applying Creamer's model of limits. Congregations practically can expand Creamer's paradigm through Reynolds' conception of "deep accessibility" and robust hospitality. He suggests that churches—as a gateway to God's loving, healing presence through everyday practices of believers—should make space for all bodies.[45] He has a fuller notion of accessibility that moves beyond architectural accommodation.

Nancy Eiesland claims that the notion of the church as a "city on a hill" has lamentably described the realities of physical inaccessibility and being socially inhospitable.[46] To combat this reality, Reynolds claims that congregations need to be cultivated "by more than generous attitudes and right beliefs. People of faith need apprenticeship into habits of care formed by a transformative spirituality of attentiveness with people with disabilities, habits that cultivate mutual partnerships of vulnerability open to the transformative power of God's grace."[47] Reynolds' model can easily be expanded beyond its practical application to persons with disabilities, to difference that marks marginalized bodies broadly.

A spirituality of attentiveness is key to *deep access*. Deep access is not superficial inclusion of persons with disability but "participation of all, which depends upon access by and for all."[48] This type of participation focuses not on "'doing for' but an equitable 'being with' in a fulsome community of vulnerable sharing life. Access is not a one-time minimalist achievement, but an ongoing welcoming accommodation to make such participation possible."[49] This is much like the congregation within rural Alabama where individuals with disabilities, addiction, and other markers of difference are part of worship and the daily functioning of the congregation. They have responsibilities within church ministry, including leadership, and are included within the ministry of accompaniment. Thus, members accompany others who are newcomers to the congregation and need resources of referral for counseling, employment, and other services to get back on their feet. The reality with such deep access and attentiveness is that there can be high turnover for leadership and those who accompany others. Sometimes, individuals will do well for months or a year and then go back to rehabilitation or back to being incarcerated, but the significance is that there is inclusion—deep access for and by all.

What is significant about deep access is its unfinished nature; it is always evolving—ever aiming for the eschatological hope of radical acceptance and full inclusion. This incomplete nature of deep access is why the practice of robust hospitality is fundamental. Robust hospitality moves beyond charitable welcome to authentic partnership between individuals.[50] Robust hospitality fosters solidarity; thus, members are attentive to differences and welcome individuals with disabilities into communion as equal, honorable, and vital members, not as needy beneficiaries of the congregation's doling out of charity.[51] Solidarity can practically take the form of activism, which includes advocacy, education to build awareness and galvanize community support, lobbying, or protest. A significant part of attentiveness is listening; acknowledging that individuals have "gifts to offer and things to say . . . is key to deep access. Listening to what is communicated is important to the process of opening further and ongoing participation in community life. It is this paying attention that is the stuff of mutual relationships of vulnerable giving and receiving, grounding worth of all."[52]

Indeed, faith communities can help modern individuals deal with the onslaught of dissatisfaction with embodiment. Congregations can minimize the effects of culturally mediated values, conditioning, and trauma by reinforcing the proposition that ". . . human nature as it is, is good, . . . we do not need to become something else, in order to reflect God's goodness; humans are already created and equipped to commune with God and others."[53] Examining how faith communities accomplish this task—not just through doctrine and transfiguring detrimental, stigmatizing narratives but through practically modeling transfigured vulnerability—is significant for fulfilling the task of being the embodied presence of Christ in society. Churches can transfigure vulnerability through practices of deep accessibility, robust hospitality, attentiveness, and solidarity, all of which build on the foundation of a reinterpretation of limits and an eschatological approach to the problem of the body in Christianity.

NOTES

1   Iris Marion Young, *Justice and the Politics of Difference* (Princeton: Princeton University Press, 1990).

2   Thomas E. Reynolds, "Invoking Deep Access: Disability beyond Inclusion in the Church," *Dialog: A Journal of Theology* 51, no. 3 (2012): 213.

3   Reynolds, "Invoking," 220.

4   Reynolds, "Invoking," 220.

5   Reynolds, "Invoking," 213.

6   See Robert H. Stein, "Is the Transfiguration (Mark 9:2–8) a Misplaced Resurrection Account?" *Journal of Biblical Literature* 95, no. 1 (1976): 79–96; see also Delbert Burkett, "The Transfiguration of Jesus,

Epiphany or Apotheosis?" *Journal of Biblical Literature* 138, no. 2 (2019): 413–32.

7   Alexander Golitzin, "'Earthly Angels and Heavenly Men': The Old Testament Pseudepigrapha, Niketas Stethatos, and the Tradition of 'Interiorized Apocalyptic' in Eastern Christian Ascetical and Mystical Literature," *Dumbarton Oaks Papers* 55 (2001): 129.

8   Stein, "Transfiguration."

9   William L. Lane, *The New International Commentary on the New Testament: The Gospel of Mark* (Grand Rapids: Eerdmans, 1974). The brightness of Jesus' garments is also interpreted as suggestive of the Shekinah, the divine presence in a pillar of fire. See Donald English, *The Message of Mark: The Mystery of Faith* (Downers Grove, Ill.: InterVarsity Press, 1992), 164.

10   Lane, *New International Commentary*, 319.

11   Lane, *New International Commentary*, 321.

12   See Kelly B. Douglas, *The Black Christ* (Maryknoll, N.Y.: Orbis Books, 1993); M. Shawn Copeland, *Enfleshing Freedom: Body, Race and Being* (Minneapolis: Fortress, 2009); James H. Cone, *God of the Oppressed* (Maryknoll, N.Y.: Orbis Books, 1975); Rosemary R. Ruether, *Sexism and God–Talk: Toward a Feminist Theology* (Boston: Beacon, 1993); Jacquelyn Grant, *White Woman's Christ, Black Woman's Jesus: Christology and Womanist Response* (Atlanta: Scholars Press, 1989).

13   Cressida J. Heyes, *Self–Transformations: Foucault, Ethics, and Normalized Bodies* (New York: Oxford University Press, 2007), 17.

14   Heyes (*Self–Transformations*, 17) criticizes normalization as defined within feminist philosophical writing as not having needed theoretical precision: "'to normalize' and its cognates are used to imply any process through which homogeneity and conformity are enforced or encouraged, or a controversial process is made to seem everyday." Heyes argues for a "complex account of normalization, as a set of mechanisms for sorting, taxonomizing, measuring, managing, and controlling populations, which both fosters conformity and generates modes of individuality, and which is at the center of an alternative picture of our history as embodied subjects."

15   Heyes, *Self–Transformations*, 17.

16   Joseph Winters, *Hope Draped in Black: Race, Melancholy, and the Agony of Progress* (Durham, N.C.: Duke University Press, 2016), 12.

17   Heyes, *Self–Transformations*. See also Deborah B. Creamer, *Disability and Christian Theology: Embodied Limits and Constructive Possibilities* (New York: Oxford University Press, 2009); Katie Geneva Cannon, Emilie Townes, and Angela D. Sims, *Womanist Theological Ethics:*

A Reader (Louisville: Westminster John Knox, 2011); Dorothy Roberts, *Fatal Invention: How Science, Politics, and Big Business Re-create Race in the Twenty-First Century* (New York: New Press, 2011); Tamura Lomax, *Jezebel Unhinged: Loosing the Black Female Body in Religion & Culture* (Durham, N.C.: Duke University Press, 2018).

18   See "Who We Are," Christian Transhumanist Association, https://www .christiantranshumanism.org/about. Some transhumanists under-stand this cultural and intellectual movement as a more radical itera-tion of secular humanism and an outgrowth of the Enlightenment (see Bostrom, "Human Genetic Enhancements"). Bostrom argues that a core transhumanist value is to explore the possibilities of posthuman exis-tence, which entails not only increased life expectancy but an enhanced "healthspan—the capacity to remain fully healthy, active and productive, both mentally and physically," (p.29) as well as cognitive and emotional capacities, including memory, reasoning, and attention, and "enhanced subjective wellbeing (joy, . . . sensual pleasures, fun, . . . excitement)" (p. 38) (Nick Bostrom, "Why I Want to Be a Posthuman When I Grow Up," in *The Transhumanist Reader: Classical and Contemporary Essays on the Science, Technology, and Philosophy of the Human Future*, ed. Max More and Nata-sha Vita-More [Malden, Mass.: Wiley-Blackwell, 2013], 29–53). Others, such as Ray Kurzweil, understand technology to be the path to exceed-ing biological limitations and reaching a state of Singularity—the belief in a situation along the path of evolution where humans will no longer witness their superiority over their creations—where machines surpass human intelligence (even emotional and moral intelligence) at an expo-nential pace. Furthermore, Singularity holds out the hope of a future state where human and machine merge, and technology will be univer-sally harnessed to solve colossal problems such as poverty or ecologi-cal devastation. See Mark O'Connell, *To Be a Machine: Adventures among Cyborgs, Utopias, Hackers, and the Futurists Solving the Modest Problem of Death* (London: Granta Publications, 2017); see also Ray Kurzweil, *The Sin-gularity Is Near* (New York: Penguin, 2006). While proponents of trans-humanism place abundant faith in the possibility of human enhance-ments in improving on what Mother Nature initiated, there is a sober acknowledgement that "transhumanism does not entail technological optimism," and there is admission of the harm that can be caused by the participation in this social experiment, such as extinction of intelligent life and "widening social inequalities or a gradual erosion of the hard-to-quantify assets that we care deeply about but tend to neglect in our daily struggle for material gain, such as meaningful human relationships and ecological diversity" (Bostrom, "Human Genetic Enhancements," 494).

19   Max More, "A Letter to Mother Nature," in More and Vita-More, *Trans-humanist Reader*.

20   See Michio Kaku, *The Future of Humanity: Terraforming Mars, Interstellar Travel, Immortality, and Our Destiny beyond Earth* (New York: Doubleday,

2018). The U.S. government has long invested in space exploration. NASA's webpage articulates the possibility of exploring space colonization: "Once the exclusive province of science fiction stories and films, the subject of space colonization has rapidly moved several steps closer to becoming a reality thanks to major advances in rocket propulsion and design, astronautics and astrophysics, robotics and medicine. The urgency to establish humanity as a multi-planet species has been re-validated by the emergence of a worldwide pandemic, one of several reasons including both natural and man-made catastrophes long espoused in the pro-colonization rhetoric." "Space Colonization," NASA, https://www.nasa.gov/centers/hq/library/find/bibliographies/space_colonization.

21   Norman Wirzba, *This Sacred Life: Humanity's Place in a Wounded World* (New York: Cambridge University Press, 2021), 44.

22   Natasha Vita-More, *Transhumanism: What Is It?* (Middletown, Del.: Self-published, 2018); "Transhumanist Manifesto," website of Natasha Vita-More, 2008, https://natashavita-more.com/transhumanist-manifesto/.

23   James Michael MacFarlane, *Transhumanism as a New Social Movement: The Techno-Centered Imagination* (Cham, Switzerland: Palgrave Macmillan, 2020).

24   Ron Cole-Turner, foreword to *Religion and the Technological Future: An Introduction to Biohacking, Artificial Intelligence, and Transhumanism*, by Calvin Mercer and Tracy J. Trothen (Cham, Switzerland: Palgrave Macmillan, 2021), ix–x.

25   Bostrom, "Human Genetic Enhancements," 493.

26   Scott MacDougall, "Bodily Communions: An Eschatological Proposal for Addressing the Christian Body Problem," *Dialog* 57 (2019): 178–85; Eboni M. Turman, "Black and Blue: Uncovering the Ecclesial Cover-up of Black Women's Bodies through a Womanist Reimagining of the Doctrine of Incarnation," in *Reimagining Doctrines: Responding to Global Gender Injustices*, ed. Grace Ji-Sun Kim and Jenny Daggers (New York: Palgrave Macmillan, 2014). See also Creamer, *Disability*; Joe Higgins, "Biosocial Selfhood: Overcoming the 'Body-Social' Problem within the Individuation of the Human Self," *Phenomenology and the Cognitive Sciences* 17 (2018): 433–54; Elisabeth Moltmann-Wendel, *I Am My Body: A Theology of Embodiment* (New York: Continuum, 1995).

27   MacDougall, "Bodily Communions," 180.

28   MacDougall, "Bodily Communions," 180. See also Moltmann-Wendel, *I Am My Body*.

29   See Eboni Marshall Turman, *Toward a Womanist Ethic of Incarnation: Black Bodies, the Black Church, and the Council of Chalcedon* (New York: Palgrave Macmillan, 2013); Janice McRandal, ed., *Sarah Coakley and*

the Future of Systematic Theology (Minneapolis: Fortress, 2016); Brian E. Daley, God Visible: Patristic Christology Revisited (Croydon, U.K.: Oxford University Press, 2018).

30 See Mark Charles and Soong-Chan Rah, Unsettling Truths: The Ongoing Dehumanizing Legacy of the Doctrine of Discovery (Downers Grove, Ill.: InterVarsity Press, 2019); Sarah Augustine, The Land Is Not Empty: Following Jesus in Dismantling the Doctrine of Discovery (Harrisonburg, Va.: Herald Press, 2021); George E. "Tink" Tinker, American Indian Liberation: A Theology of Sovereignty (Maryknoll, N.Y.: Orbis Books, 2008); see also Luis N. Rivera-Pagan, A Violent Evangelicalism: The Political and Religious Conquest of the Americas (Louisville: John Knox, 1992).

31 See Kelly B. Douglas, The Black Christ (Maryknoll, N.Y.: Orbis Books, 1993); M. Shawn Copeland, Enfleshing Freedom: Body, Race and Being (Minneapolis: Fortress, 2009); Cone, God of the Oppressed; Ruether, Sexism; Grant, White Woman's Christ.

32 Lisa Cahill, "Kingdom and Cross: Christian Moral Community and the Problem of Suffering," Interpretation 50, no. 2 (1996): 156.

33 Cahill, "Kingdom," 155.

34 Reynolds, "Invoking," 222.

35 Creamer, Disability, 116.

36 Creamer, Disability, 116

37 Creamer, Disability, 93.

38 Creamer, Disability, 93.

39 Creamer, Disability, 93 (emphasis original).

40 Creamer, Disability, 94–119.

41 Creamer, Disability, 94–119.

42 Creamer, Disability, 117.

43 Creamer, Disability, 117.

44 Creamer, Disability, 117.

45 Reynolds, "Invoking," 212.

46 Eiesland, Disabled God, 20.

47 Reynolds, "Invoking," 222.

48 Reynolds, "Invoking," 221.

49 Reynolds, "Invoking," 221.

50 Letty M. Russell, Just Hospitality: God's Welcome in a World of Difference (Louisville: Westminster John Knox, 2009).

51 Russell, Just Hospitality.

52 Reynolds, "Invoking," 221.

53 Bioenhancement Propositions Table, pp. 9–10 above.

7

THE LAME TO WALK AND THE DEAF FEAR

Why It Pays for Surveillance Capitalism
to Exploit the Disabled

Brian Brock

THIBAULT AND HIS EXOSKELETON

On the fourth of October, 2019, at Clinatec, a private biomedical research center in Grenoble, France, a man publicly known as "Thibault" stood up and walked. At the time a twenty-eight-year-old tetraplegic, Thibault had previously broken his neck in a fall from a fourth-floor balcony during a party.[1] Through an intense regime of experimental surgery, therapy, and technology, the sensors on the surface of his brain were now sufficiently sensitive to allow him to move all four of his paralyzed limbs by way of a mind-controlled exoskeleton suit. Awed by his experience, Thibault compared himself to the first man on the moon and expressed special appreciation for regaining his upright bodily stance: "I had forgotten that I used to be taller than a lot of people in the room. It was very impressive."[2]

The researchers in charge of the experimental procedure were not only technically cutting-edge but media savvy. On the day of the announcement that Thibault was walking again, the global media had all the glossy images and expert quotes they needed to broadcast the feat far and wide. The announcement of an event that had taken place behind the closed doors of a scientific lab was announced along with a series of photos of Thibault strapped into a remarkably glossy-looking exoskeleton in a suspiciously color-coordinated bioscience facility. A short and distinctly less impressive and aesthetically harmonious video of him in motion was also available. The articles that flooded the news-scape invariably invoked the scientific-progress-gives-us-hope narrative, and for many the media blitz clearly worked. As one person commented, "Always remember: For all the stories about stupidity and ones that make you feel like society is 'circling the drain,' advances like these are still being made by our most brilliant minds."[3]

As a public relations feat, Thibault's walking far surpassed previous unveilings such as the one that opened the 2014 World Cup in Brazil. There twenty-nine-year-old Juliano Pinto, a paraplegic man, used his neural interface to flex one leg to kick the first ball into play. His glitzy but primitive mechanical suit had been produced by researchers from Duke University's Center for Neuroengineering in cooperation with other private companies.[4] As of 2019, people in the United Kingdom were more aware of the various displays of the paraplegic American Paralympian Jennifer French standing up from her wheelchair by activating muscle-controlling neural implants.[5] All of these stories play to a well-entrenched cultural script that features the restoration of the power to stand and walk as self-evidently attractive.[6]

One of the watershed moments in the establishment of this public narrative came in the late 1990s when the Hollywood star Christopher Reeve very publicly announced his determination to walk again after having been paralyzed in a horse-riding accident. This narrative arguably reached a new cultural ascendency with the release of *Avatar*, the highest-grossing Hollywood film to that date. The main character in this story is a paraplegic man with a neural interface that allows him to inhabit a biological full-body prosthesis, into which his mind is eventually fully merged and his broken human body discarded.[7] The medical researchers who fitted Thibault in his exoskeleton transparently positioned their work within this cultural narrative, asserting, "The exoskeleton is a biometric anthropomorphic neuroprosthesis and is possibly the best solution to totally compensate for the impairment in a patient with tetraplegia."[8]

In this chapter, I approach familiar debates about the relation of therapeutic treatments to technological enhancements of the human from the point of view of disabled life as understood in Christian disability theology. In Christian theology, finitude and limitation are not a curse but welcomed. The majority of this paper is devoted to describing in detail exactly how we modern citizens of the developed West embody a repudiation of this claim. I will tell the story of one biomedical intervention in order to concretely display what I mean with this claim. The question "what does it mean to be human?" is one that we incrementally answer in the acts of everyday life. Being human is not a theory, a concept. Being human is a task, one we answer with every act, since, as Luther so often taught, there is no way of living or dying that is religiously neutral.[9]

The aim of this description is to show how the form of humanity we are currently living out is one in which we interact with one another as streams of information. The hopes of a capitalistic society to secure peace through material wealth converge to form a society-wide consensus that the future is best secured by developing better and more certain ways to mine and so control the information each person generates, just by living. What is well known is that we are increasingly becoming data shadows to be manipulated by business and government.[10] What this essay further explicates is how this cultural consensus, this belief in the importance of wealth and security, ends up exploiting people with disabilities.

This line of argument is in part a pushback against the consensus that has emerged among theologically oriented medical ethicists that the distinction between medical therapies and enhancements are no longer conceptually useful for distinguishing between research into new treatments and biotechnologies.[11] I will show that entirely abandoning the therapy-enhancement distinction abandons people with disabilities to the depredations of market economics. What are popularly called therapeutic medical interventions, in which the human body is altered in order to reduce suffering or restore lost functioning, are theologically and ethically uncontentious. In principle Christians can and in many cases should embrace medicine, surgery, and pharmaceutical treatments as a way of receiving their bodies from God with gratitude. But licit medical therapies can be misused, and those who are developing what are popularly called enhancements today are developing forms of medical procedure that aim to improve well-functioning bodies. The misuse of therapy and the desire to improve the well-functioning human body is the focus of this paper. The main part of my proposal is the suggestion that the therapy–enhancement distinction is a barrier to the designs of industry and political leaders to achieve the widespread use of human enhancements—enhancements of what we today think of as perfectly normally functioning bodies. The alteration of these bodies is unthinkable for most today, so powerful agents in developed societies today have good reason to introduce them as therapeutic techniques—a ploy in which disabled lives are used as pawns in an indefensible manner.

A brief final comment unveils how such desires must be understood as springing from a theological deformation. The dreams of transcending human finitude and vulnerability that have generated technologies like Thibault's exoskeleton express transhumanist desires to overcome the body that have no sense of what it means to live with mortal bodies in the power of the resurrecting Spirit. The transhumanist hopes to transcend the body are, fundamentally, the hope to master materiality. It is the modern hope to overcome and control nature writ large. Christian hope, in contrast, is one that embraces death as a constitutive reality for creaturely bodies and seeks a way of living in mutually upbuilding communion with one's own body and with other creatures. This affirmation of the goodness of the material world positions humans as hoping to be transformed into beings capable of living at peace—sustainably—in a material world that Christians confess is good and sufficient to fulfill the needs of every creature. The thoroughgoing commitment of transhumanists to imminent reality being all there is leads them to discount richer forms of hoping, making them unable to hope for genuine renewal of the individual's mind and social sensibility. Desiring to remake the body, transhumanists cannot imagine the more sweeping remaking of human self–understanding that is fundamental to Christian hope.

A Closer Look at Public Attitudes to Ameliorating Disability

Most debates about the therapy–enhancement divide in the academic discourses of philosophical and theological ethics barely engage the moral landscape in which debates about human enhancement and the posthuman are taking place. A brief summary of a report compiled on behalf of the Royal Society on public attitudes helpfully illuminates attitudes of the general public in the United Kingdom to neural interfaces in the nation. This survey indicates how most people understand the relationship between enhancement technologies and disability, at least as they did in 2019.[12] This social scientific research relied on a large and representatively diverse group of respondents. Focus-group discussions began probing people's opinions about therapeutic use of neural interfaces by showing them examples of people in wheelchairs being able to stand up with help from cortical implants, or people with Parkinson's disease using a switch to halt their tremors by activating a wire that stimulated the affected region deep in their brain. The leading-edge example of a successful neural interface is the cochlear implant to treat hearing loss.[13] Yet those who described the benefits of this neural interface often did so in ways that indicated a desire to eliminate disability. "Anything to help the future generations overcome disability is a good thing," as one cochlear implant user group respondent put it.[14]

Perhaps one of the most ironic discoveries of the report is that the desire to create a more inclusive society is the most significant driver of the desire to eradicate disability. One group in Glasgow, for instance, remarked:

> Your neutral interfaces essentially are taking away the disabilities. They're creating a more level playing field where everyone essentially becomes equal. When everyone's equal and you get rid of the marginalisation so that people aren't outsiders due to their disabilities, as perhaps they would have been otherwise.[15]

A group in Sheffield stated the eliminationist subtext of this remark more bluntly: "Everybody will now be created equal. . . . There will be no disabilities anymore. Everybody will be included. Everybody who now currently can't speak, will be able to engage fully in a full, productive life."[16]

Wide swaths of the British public seem to agree that the eradication of disability is a worthwhile scientific aim. One driver of this view is the belief that to remain socially connected in modern developed societies, people need to be independently mobile:

> People affected by Parkinson's disease predicted in their discussions that in 20 years' time any neurological and neuro degenerative conditions, such as multiple sclerosis, Parkinson's and Alzheimer's disease could be fully treated by neural implants.

Others in the dialogue workshops spoke of their optimism for a future where there is no need for mobility assistance devices because of advances in Mollii suits and equivalent therapeutic devices. [In the words of one Glasgow respondent], "We believe that (by 2050) there will no longer be a use for wheelchairs or mobility assistance due to the suit being able to build muscle back into people's body and the spinal nerve connection. We could eradicate everyone's mobility issues in 30 years' time."[17]

Respondents felt that any technology that could increase independence was promising, because "current community structures very rarely allow for sufficient informal support for those who are relying on others for their basic care. [As one respondent in Glasgow remarked], 'Society has become so fragmented now. . . . This gives people a choice to potentially support themselves.'"[18] The dream of the eradication of disabilities rests on deeply interwoven and also contradictory desires for community and supportive relationships as well as the aspiration for mobility and financial independence.

Some cochlear implant users felt that improved neural link technologies promise to remove individuals altogether from the stigmatized category of the disabled. If this is achievable, it will be because the technology has succeeded in hiding itself. As authors of the report note, "Several participants in the Cochlear Implant User Group talked about the new development in cochlear implants which will be fully internal and controlled by a mobile phone. This was liked for taking away the stigma of an external hearing device."[19] Even those with the most successful therapeutic types of neural interfaces, cochlear implants, felt keenly aware that the very devices that were eliminating their disability were not in fact curing, but only ameliorating, it. This cohort of technology users was no doubt aware that cochlear implants do not restore anything like "normal" hearing. They worried more about the cloaking of their prosthetic technologies in order to relieve them of being stigmatized as disabled[20] than they did about these prostheses seamlessly[21] restoring—let alone enhancing—their capacity to hear.

Intriguingly, the study also drew attention to the ways in which brain-computer interfaces might help disabled people and in so doing also burnish the reputation of technology itself: "Some participants saw the application of neural interfaces solving some of the world's most intractable medical problems as a hugely positive contribution to the narrative around technology in general. They thought that neural interfaces that could restore movement to those who are paralyzed or sight to those who are blind could help to rebalance the tech narrative that to date has been dominated by large social media companies and their use of data and artificial intelligence to influence our behavior."[22] Some might see the polyvalence about who benefits from these technologies as a win–win situation, for, in staving off widely shared dystopian worries about technology, the technological project itself was being rehabilitated and with it the tech companies bringing these technologies to the marketplace. In the words of one London participant, "It develops a positive narrative for technology. Not every tech gets a bad record but more from the media it gets quite negative."[23]

One widespread point of consensus across geography and demographic differences was a sense that a widespread use of neural implants is likely to cause a major shift in public understandings of injury, disability, and "normal" human performance:

> The more conditions and disabilities that are treatable, the fewer disabled people there will be. Although that will mean that fewer people will be defined by their disability, many participants felt strongly that this can lead to a society in which people become more intolerant and less appreciative of diversity. This was seen as an undesirable future, as it may lead to a greater stigmatisation of those with untreatable disability or conditions. Participants said that this throws up ethical questions, e.g. who decides which disabilities will be prioritised for neural implant treatment and why. Conversations with cochlear implant users showed that some had encountered resistance in the deaf community against their decision to accept a cochlear implant. They said that in the deaf community, identity is shaped by communicating in other ways than is the societal norm. In a similar vein, discussions about the use of EEG for education led to a view in the dialogue that this type of non-medical neural implant can potentially contribute to the creation of a subset of an ever more uniform society that is stigmatised and at risk of being bullied.[24]

The Royal Society study also found that these negative impacts on disabled people's lives were coupled with further worries about nontherapeutic neural interfaces being implanted in otherwise healthy subjects. Suspicion abounds that nonmedical uses of neural implants are frivolous, worrying, or both. Many of these worries followed lines well-travelled in dystopian science fiction—that such technologies might lead to physical or mental laziness, or to big business controlling people's minds. Interestingly, these British respondents also considered it irresponsible to develop any of these technologies—even for therapeutic uses—if they were not to be widely available. The development of a two-tiered society of haves and have-nots lies behind this worry, as well as a firm commitment to equality in health care.

In this cultural context, it becomes clearer why the Clinatec media blitz around Thibault's walking is not an add-on to the "hard" science but intrinsic to the further success of the work going on in this biotech context. As long as public opinion is dominated by worries about neural technologies, the companies and governments who are funding them have little hope of recovering their investment and bringing them into widespread use.

The Adventus of Neural Interfaces: Will We Be Ready?

Insiders in industry and science generally assume public resistance to placing neural implants in healthy people will disappear. The question is not *whether* that will happen, but *when*.[25] The next three sections will indicate why we do not need to imagine that this certainty about the inevitability of widespread neural interface use is somehow being driven by a transhumanist avant-garde who know that the perfecting of such technologies is a necessary step to transcending the human as depicted in movies like *Avatar*. Tracing the technological evolution currently underway in developed societies indicates why the pressure to develop neural interfaces is more likely to grow than subside. Strong imperatives in this direction are already hardwired into our newly "wired" daily lives, economics, and political orders.

No consumer object in the history of the world has been so quickly and so universally adopted as the smartphone, and we have only begun to intuit what this change means for our societies, our psyches, and our ways of organizing the world.[26] Most of the human population has already become reliant on uninterrupted connection to the internet to accomplish daily goals. The smartphone was the first and most visible harbinger of a world called "the internet of things," which can be seen as the extension of the networked human into more and more active devices. Wearable biometric sensors like Fitbit and Apple Watch are already well known, as is their aim to offer more of the individual physical body and its functions as computationally available information. Having utilized biometric monitoring to optimize our own bodies, the utility of applying the same logic to make the many bodies that make up society more efficient appears self-evident. A "smart" home is a home where you do not have to think about adjusting the thermostat to stay comfortable, where a word can dim the lights or cue the music, and from which our every daily need becomes accessible to the corporations like Amazon designed to seamlessly meet them. The smart city is a citywide version of the same—where the traffic lights automatically adjust according to traffic levels, where police are always present when suspicious people congregate, where rental rates for shop space can be precisely calibrated according to pedestrian footfall, and where energy use and waste disposal can be anticipated and so Pareto-optimized. The humming hive that is human society is constantly generating information that can be captured and fed into the internet so that it can be continuously and algorithmically optimized. And this is a world in which we cannot participate without surrendering vast amounts of data.[27]

The information generated by all these wired devices about what we want, what we are doing, and how we communicate with each other is the raw material of our generation's new gold rush, which promises to remake our societies as fundamentally as did the discovery of fossil fuels. Shoshana Zuboff has recently documented this startling claim by asking what might be learned from the fact that the most spectacular wealth creators of the last decades have all been internet and technology companies. In the world in which everything is wired, information becomes the new currency. This is why we must understand Western developed nations to be entering a new era of capitalism she calls "surveillance capitalism." Once a critical mass of sensors and computing power are in place, prediction becomes the new and central economic and political imperative. This theme has been explored in fiction,[28] but contemporary sociological research has substantiated that the central driver of this evolution is an obvious development from previous understandings of marketing. Whereas once marketers promised to change behavior while not being able to prove that they had, in the new information economy the only change that matters is the change that produces tangible and testable real-time movements in human behavior. This is obviously a technique as suitable for moving consumers as for controlling national citizens.[29] This is the richest vein for which the new gold rush is aiming.[30]

The entire business model of companies like Facebook, Google, and Amazon is organized around generating ever deeper and broader information flows around consumer activity by harvesting and synchronizing information flows from across widely different platforms. Companies built on the techniques of data mining need to know what we talk about at breakfast, how much time we spend commuting to work, what we like in our refrigerators, and what we do for relaxation in our living rooms. The aim is to predict what we will do next. They need to understand the ebb and flow of our moods, what we lie about, and what we search for when no one is looking in order to effectively steer us toward the consumption that can be predicted and so capitalized. The gold of the new economy is knowledge of reality, the reality of our desires. "The aim of this undertaking is not to impose behavioral norms, such as conformity or obedience, but rather to produce behavior that reliably, definitively and certainly leads to desired commercial results. The research director of Gartner, the well-respected business advisory and research firm, makes the point . . . that mastery of the 'internet of things' will serve as 'a key enabler in the transformation of business models from "guaranteed levels of performance" to "*guaranteed outcomes*".'"[31]

The holy grail of this new economy is to know the unconscious mind, and here again we meet a story in which the therapy of disability seems to be functioning as a Trojan horse for something very different. Professor Rosalind Picard, of the MIT Media Lab, is one of the pioneers of what has come to be called "affective computing," the automated sensing and processing of emotional states based on gauging a user's facial micro-expressions. The goal for such programs is to render both conscious and unconscious behavior as coded and calculable information streams. Picard's basic scientific work aimed to help autistic children develop skills in emotional communication and led to the development of computer games capable of fostering this emotional learning. Picard herself had some foreboding about what the tech giants and governments might do with this technology, understanding the strength of their incentives to sell us things in moments of emotional vulnerability or to seek to manipulate or control the emotions of a population. As it turns out, her fears were well placed, and only twenty years after the publication of Picard's research, a leading market research firm predicted that the "affective computing market" would grow from $9.35 billion in 2015 to $53.98 billion in 2021, a growth rate of nearly 35 percent driven almost exclusively by the marketing and advertising sector.[32]

Picard's story helps us to see how the aims of researchers to offer disabled people empowering therapies are vastly overshadowed by the interests of agents driven by commercial aims. Picard and her protégé at MIT, Rana el Kaliouby, used their research to build a machine system they called Mind-Reader, which they initially trained to recognize emotions by using paid actors to mimic specific emotional responses and characteristic facial gestures. Soon the pair were overwhelmed by inquiries from major corporations who wanted to use the technology to measure their customers' emotional responses. MIT encouraged Picard and Kaliouby to spin off a startup company around their technology, called Affectiva, of which Picard soon discovered herself elbowed out of control. The company boomed under the leadership of Kaliouby, who took it to venture capitalists and does business with thirty-two Fortune 100 companies and fourteen hundred global brands. Kaliouby now imagines that "pervasive 'emotional scanning' will come to be as taken for granted as a 'cookie' planted in your computer to track your online browsing. After all, those cookies once stirred outrage, and now they inundate every online move."[33]

It is not the therapeutic but the economic promise of these technologies that becomes most obvious to close observers such as Danielle Carr, a historian of these technologies: "Real-time information about neural activity is currently one of the hardest forms of data to acquire: everyone has a phone, but very few people have neural implants. This is why patients with Deep Brain Stimulation implants are treated as precious resources by scientific researchers; they often work simultaneously with multiple research teams running experiments in which the brain data gleaned by the device can be coupled with behavioral data. By combining different forms of data—the sort of information your phone collects, for example, and cortex activity—both sets become more meaningful."[34] In the midst of such a gold rush, however long it lasts, the culturally assessed stock price of those with the right disabilities will be soaring. The economic incentives here are so strong that it is hard to see how even the highest aspirations to serve those with disabilities will not be co-opted, as happened to Picard. The time may have come to relinquish our qualms and embrace the future of Western society as announced by the paralyzed American Adam Gorlitsky: "Either you adapt or you die."[35] Paralyzed from the waist down, Gorlitsky trained in his ReWalk exoskeleton to compete with a British man for the title of the fastest paralyzed man to complete a marathon. "In a weird way," he says, "it's a good time to be paralyzed."[36] The leaders of Silicon Valley's science and industry elites could not agree more, and from their perspective his message has the advantage of being culturally attractive. Gorlitsky's story proved the perfect leading episode in the tellingly titled video series *Freethink Superhuman*.

Public Opinion and Therapeutic Intervention

It is now becoming clearer that the role allocated to people with disabilities is positioned by the technological and economic imperative to develop neural interface technologies. As we have seen, significant sectors of the general public are worried about the ethical implications of neural interfaces but see therapeutic uses as defensible. Having surveyed a wide spectrum of British citizens, the independent (meaning not industry sponsored) authors of the Royal Society study project surveyed in the previous section concluded that the general public has "strong support for neural interfaces in situations where they enable patients to recover something that has been lost due to injury or a medical condition; but less support for the technology when it is used to enhance functions such as memory, concentration or physical skills among healthy people."[37] We can be sure that Alim Louis Benabid understood that this was the crucial moral landscape in which his neural interface research that culminated in Thibault's exoskeleton would stand or fall. As one of the professors at Grenoble leading the project and the lead author of the study published in *Lancet Neurology*, he no doubt has much riding on its success, also being the founder and executive board president of the biomedical firm Clinatec.[38] It is now evident why he was so insistent that his aim in this research is to develop a therapeutic technology, distancing himself from any insinuation that such technologies were about human enhancement: "This isn't about turning man into machine but about responding to a medical problem. . . . We're talking about 'repaired man,' not 'augmented man.'"[39]

One reason for Benabid to underline the therapeutic nature of Thibault's treatment was that the legal hurdles would have been much higher (and the PR benefit much lower) were such invasive surgery undertaken on an otherwise healthy person. In offering such treatments to a disabled person, Benabid continues a long tradition of building the edifice of modern medicine on the back of those with questionable capacity to consent to it.[40] Even if the technology works and begins to be used more widely, such technologies will remain legally risky in undermining the functioning of a formerly healthy body. This remains the case even though almost all nontherapeutic medical treatments started off as therapeutic—cosmetic surgery was initially restorative, growth hormone developed for those who had a HGH deficiency, and so forth—but where these produce negative medical outcomes, the sense of patient outrage is understandable and risky for the doctor. On these grounds, both the level of biomedical research ethics and contemporary malpractice law, a working therapy–enhancement distinction remains an important part of the apparatus sustaining a just society. Once the technology is proved in the context of therapeutic uses, it fundamentally shifts the parameters of public debates about more widespread uses of neural interfaces. A chasm of cultural resistance and prejudice against these technologies must be crossed if the miniscule numbers of early adopters of these technologies in high-tech settings is to be diffused more generally through society, so catalyzing entirely new ways of performing a host of traditional kinds of work. These are crucial issues for investors and industry leaders since neural interfaces are disruptive technologies.

The question of how to persuade the wider populace to accept these technologies is exercising many of the best minds in industry, and the story always begins with the promise of medical treatments. Consider the roadmap proposed by Professor Tim Denison, professor of neurotechnology at the University of Oxford:

> To help focus investment, neural interface technologies could benefit from an industry roadmap. Roadmaps can help guide the development of applications in a manner that meet [sic] the balanced requirements for successful translation, including economics. One historical example of successful application of platform deployment is provided by the innovator, Alfred E Mann. Mann's group developed a 16-channel cochlear implant for the hearing impaired. From this core stimulator, they expanded to a 16-channel spinal cord stimulator for chronic pain. Finally, they built a prototype of what would become the Argus retinal prosthesis using the same core building blocks. Common platforms can help to lower the marginal investment cost for exploring new ideas. . . . While the 16-channel retinal implant was useful as a prototype, it was upgraded to a 64-channel system before commercial translation as a humanitarian device exemption.[41]

Denison's three-step movement to "commercial translation" cannot get started without the development of medical applications. His proposed progression begins with the development of technologies capable of neuromodulation (treating Parkinson's disease, epilepsy, or chronic pain; assistive technologies; or mental health monitoring), followed by those that can be developed in consumer electronics (enhanced gaming, neurofeedback, and meditation assistance), and culminating in medicalized products offered to the consumer, which he labels as neuromarketed products for cognitive enhancement (memory, alertness, sleep quality, and academic performance enhancements).[42] The tension people feel between the hope for mastery and the hope for meaningful personal integrity is being met with the response: "But perhaps you could hope that these technologies might only enhance the 'real' you, since they will only augment those aspects of you that you already value?"

The Prospectors in the Neural Gold Rush

Elon Musk is another keen investor in brain-machine interfacing, not wanting to be bypassed by the medical technologists at Clinatec,

Duke, and other biotech companies on a lucrative technological market. Musk has had some success with his robotic device for implanting brain-reading microfibers on the living brains of rats, monkeys, and pigs.[43] Perhaps unsurprisingly, Musk tends to find it harder than a full-time medical researcher like Benabid to present his project as a genuinely therapeutic intervention, his language falling into his native engineer-problem-solving idiom that sits at some distance from the hospital. At one live Neuralink event, for example, he emphasized that Neuralink technology would be able to treat a wide variety of spinal neurological conditions, including seizures, paralysis, brain damage, and depression. "These can all be solved with an implantable neural link," said Musk. "The neurons are like wiring, and you kind of need an electronic thing to solve an electronic problem." The company's aim is to "build an incredibly powerful brain-machine interface, a device with the power to handle lots of data, that can be inserted in a relatively simple surgery. Its short-term goal is to build a device that can help people with specific health conditions."[44]

What is important for our purposes is Neuralink's explicit admission that therapy is the "short-term goal" in the development of neural implant technology. Having worked with animals, Musk makes usefully explicit what I have suggested is only a tactical engagement in serving disabled people and people with "specific health conditions." Even if we grant Musk has noble desires to better the lives of disabled and mentally ill people,[45] we have already seen the reasons why those good intentions offer little protection against "long-term" market imperatives. Making quadriplegics walk will never be lucrative business, unless we see a radical reevaluation of the levels of investment in making this happen than we see today. (For instance, a friend in the Aberdeen rehabilitation and mobility service, which cares for some nine thousand patients in the region, told me that only a fraction are offered the "platinum" service of a powered wheelchair. Most are offered techniques of relational and practical empowerment to help them to live more peacefully with their new condition.) The distance between what these technologies are supposed to promise and what they actually can deliver in the ethico-political landscape of our present suggests that if Musk has made a contribution to the public discussion of neural implantations, it is not by making an advance in science but by performing a bit of science theater to legitimate the idea that the technology is capable of offering some sort of broad-based promise to those disenfranchised by their disabilities. As Danielle Carr observes:

> Of all the wild speculations Elon Musk made during the Neuralink launch, the most accurate prediction was his quip that the device is "sort of like if your phone went in your brain." "Sort of like," indeed: Neuralink *is* like a phone in that it is yet another machine built for generating data. While the device does not represent a major advance in brain-machine interfaces, and the pipeline for applications beyond movement disorders is at best decades long, what Neuralink *does* offer is an opportunity to harvest data about the brain and couple it to the kinds of data about our choices and behaviors that are already being collected all the time. The device is best understood not as a rupture with the past, but as an intensification of the forms of surveillance and data accumulation that have come to define our everyday lives.[46]

One detail worth further examination is Musk's open avowal that some of the treatments he is imagining are ones that use neural links not in order for humans to control machines but so that machines can alter the mind, as in ameliorating depression (it should be noted that this aim is far more difficult and aspirational than physical movement, given that mental states are much less localized in one part of the brain).[47] Many of the uses of these technologies that we might see in the next decade or less move in this computer-to-brain direction, at least if business strategists' predictions are accurate. Some relatively noninvasive brain-computer interfaces could, for instance, warn you when your attention is wandering, adjust the lighting in an office if the occupant is becoming stressed, or disable a company car if the driver is too drowsy. Some companies already have a dashboard that allows workers and managers to monitor the attention levels of their colleagues. Industry insiders predict that many of the more dangerous jobs in developed economies will eventually require brain-function monitoring of this type. More actively, these technologies can also enable people to control a PowerPoint presentation or Excel spreadsheet by a thought command. It is likely that "passthoughts" will be developed as a stronger biometric alternative to computer passwords.[48]

Western militaries have long dreamed of neuroenhancements, with neuroimplantation being a central focus of research. Military researchers hope to develop external suits to improve physical capacities of soldiers, not least because of the cultural legibility of superpower-granting exoskeletons like the comic book hero Iron Man. The need for exoskeletons to closely follow the movement of a soldier's body drives the quest of researchers to find new ways to more closely link the computer and the body, whether through central or peripheral nervous system interfaces.[49] Research is also ongoing on a range of other defense uses, such as to direct drones or other remotely operated vehicles, and it is here where we can see an obvious proximity of the therapeutic and military use of neuroimplants.[50] The most pressing reason why brain-computer interfaces are inevitable from the perspective of modern militaries is that the amount of information that needs to be immediately processed on the wired battlefield is overwhelming, which explains why the "Brain-Interface Project" is the most lavishly funded research program in the DARPA bioengineering program.[51]

Technology companies like Ekso Bionics (suppliers of paralyzed marathoner Adam Gorlitsky's exoskeleton) are also counting on the appeal of exoskeletons and other neuroprosthetics to people with limb paralysis and money to spend for high-end prosthetics. Even though the technologies of neuroimplantation and exoskeleton prostheses are at highly variable levels of development, the promise of alleviation or the insinuation of a cure for paralysis remains a powerful marketing draw for those with able minds but bodies they cannot control.[52] Those with paraplegic and tetraplegic family members tell me that they are astonished by the frequency that family members and friends send them stories of the miraculous power and promise of such healing technologies.

THE POLITICAL UTILITY OF DISABILITY ANXIETY

Popular anxiety about disability is politically useful to governing elites. The crux of the story I have told thus far turns on the attempt to move popular attitudes regarding disability toward a greater acceptance of wider deployments of neural interfaces to healthy people. We can now see that the particular problem in this specific case is that the general public is unsettled by precisely those uses that those developing neural interface technologies foresee them being used for. Because people are nervous about the suggestion that they need wires implanted in their brains in order to better control computers or to work more efficiently, those determined to profit from their development need to find a way to convince the public that it is ethically laudable to develop these technologies. We can go so far as to say that researchers and political strategists are vulnerably dependent on having a public that takes it as axiomatic truth that quadriplegics want to walk, just as those with other neurological conditions are desperate to be technologically healed. As long as there is widespread public support for the alleviation of illnesses and disabilities by any means, potential exists for breaking down people's fears about wider diffusion of the technology. Certainty about the rightness of eliminating disability is perfectly suited to bypass ethical qualms in the popular mind about a technology that pushes toward applications to extend beyond normal human capacity.

In fact, there have been recurrent deployments in modern developed nations of the fear of disability to produce political movement in populations. During the nineteenth century, for example, people with Down syndrome played this role. The doctor whose name was the source of the label "Down syndrome," John Langdon Down, based his theory of the condition on nineteenth-century racial classification systems. By classifying "idiots," Down was able to bolster his professional authority as an expert in the causes and development of the condition, and then shape public policy toward his preferred solution, institutional segregation. The power of anxiety was at the heart of his analysis. His theory was elegantly, even simplistically, focused on anxiety. Down syndrome was caused by maternal anxiety during pregnancy, and the presence of people with Down syndrome caused people anxiety. By regularly highlighting the anxiety of parents of children with Down syndrome, Down bolstered his case for his preferred political proposal: institutions in which people with disparate intellectual capacities could be kept away from the general populace. Thus, as Stacy Simplican has observed, "Down helped craft an anxiety of disability that arises between people due to incommensurate capacities. Down prom-ised to ease this anxiety by first adding precision to the identifica-tion of idiots, then segregating them accordingly."[53] More recently, the high visibility of Down syndrome and public anxiety about the condition has again been harnessed to foster public acceptance of another technology initially viewed with popular skepticism: prena-tal screening technologies—technologies designed from the outset with the aim in mind of eliminating people with Down syndrome, but also promising to eliminate other congenital conditions.[54]

The ground we have covered now makes it clear that there are substantial ethical questions at stake around neural implant tech-nologies, and they are ones with direct links to the management of modern developed nation-states in the economic, policing, and medical domains. The COVID-19 pandemic has provided ample displays of the capacity of nation-states to deploy their legal power to confine populations to their homes, and their financial and industrial might to quickly develop new vaccines and deliver them to whole populations. As in previous eras, in such an emer-gency condition, governing authorities are often granted the power to rewrite laws and rules, without the usual safeguards. The more existentially threatening the emergency, the more obviously licit this rewriting of convention and law becomes, as Carl Schmitt so influentially argued. This happens differently, at once more sub-tly and invasively, in a bureaucratically managed surveillance state. Whereas infected citizens in previous eras could be walled off in a part of the city, essentially to die, our society need not physically segregate bodies but only to institute highly intricate track-and-trace systems, systems that are doubly useful in promising the constant goal of the wired society: hot-spot policing. In the pro-cess, laboriously constructed but tenuously balanced privacy pro-tections are almost instantly swept away.

The basic political problem presented by the technologies of neuroimplantation is that the lowest-risk procedures, such as deep brain simulation, are minimally invasive and so not very risky but are effective at altering the brain, not using the brain to control a com-puter.[55] More contacts are needed with disparate parts of the brain if the flow of electrical information is to be reversed and to become rich enough to be usable for directing computers. Thibault's sensors had to be large in order to allow more sensors to contact a greater number of points on the surface of the brain. Here we have the catch-22 for those who wish to see widespread neural interfaces, because very few of us would consent to have two five-centimeter holes drilled in our skulls. But for the elite who clearly see the great windfall that widespread use of neural interfaces promises, emergency cases such as Thibault's paralysis present themselves as an opportunity to dissolve the current legal and social resistance to such alterations of the human body. To achieve this end may occasionally demand that social anxiety about certain states of disabled life be increased through public messaging, as it has historically been in the past. What matters is that cases are found in which the unthinkable can be attempted. Once the technique has been safely accomplished, and its utility made publicly manifest through the usual media channels, an idea that had once been unthinkable can be presented in terms that the masses might find more acceptable. It soon will be forgotten that a technique first developed to serve a subpopulation that the public pities ought now be considered for its continuing profitability and usefulness.

So do techniques developed to "cure" a human condition that is widely feared become the occasion for the emergence of a new normal. We are used to the story of disabled lives being segregated, sequestered, and even remade for the good of the managed society.[56] What I am highlighting is the incorporation of disabled lives into a posthuman story about the good life for humans. Here disabled lives are not hidden away but rendered meaningful as a gateway to a new social order, and so meaningful, at least for a moment.

On Paralysis and Exoskeletons

What popular feel-good articles and science-fiction films tend to hide away is the intense labor and great expense entailed in attempts at medical restoration of paralyzed limbs. Anyone who has spent any time around someone with a paralyzed limb or limbs will be aware that, relatively quickly after the loss of nerve control, a limb will contract and atrophy, to the extent that bending joints becomes difficult and painful. This is why putting a tetraplegic upright and forcing their limbs to move in a walking motion will never be the medically optimal or cost-efficient way to improve mobility.

The details provided in the official scientific report of Thibault's big walk make this point abundantly clear. We learn that his five meters of self-propelled locomotion while suspended by a ceiling track was the culmination of two years of preparation.[57] Thibault is paralyzed from his C5 vertebrae and had been only one of two who qualified for the research project, and the only one whose brain implants had worked as planned. The central technical innovation was a five-centimeter round disk with highly sensitive electric sensors on its surface. Only slightly thicker than the depth of the skull, this sensor was positioned outside the protective membrane around the brain, above the motor cortex in both of the brain's hemispheres. The innovation is this placement of the sensing apparatus on the membrane of the brain rather than inserting wires through that membrane, which tends to provoke immune responses. Two five-centimeter holes had to be cut into Thibault's skull in order for the sensors to be fitted, which are meant to remain there permanently. All previous approaches have attempted to avoid such large excisions of healthy skull bone, with the previous wire-implanting approaches requiring drilling only small holes in the skull. The first patient who had these new sensors implanted was left with two large holes in his skull when the malfunctioning units had to be removed, a not-insignificant negative outcome.

The academic article on the procedure Thibault underwent exposes what is artfully hidden in popular articles: this is a highly expensive research protocol and would only function in a resource-intensive environment. Surgeons are needed to implant the sensors, physiologists to stretch atrophying muscles, computer technicians to monitor and update software, and engineers to oversee the mechanical aspects of the exoskeleton. This is many orders of magnitude more expensive and complex than the implantation of a single wire into the brain of a patient suffering from Parkinson's disease, which this more complex sensor only superficially resembles. And even with these much more sensitive sensors implanted, the notion that they provided enough neural feedback to allow Thibault actually to walk remains a bit of a sleight of hand: his exoskeleton is still tethered to a track on the ceiling of his lab, and it is clear from the videos released that very little weight rests on his feet. He is "walking" only in the sense that his limbs are making the basic motions of the walking gait, initiated if not controlled by his mind. He is in no sense standing on his own two feet, and we are a long way from the sensors having the bandwidth, for instance, to allow Thibault to catch himself should he trip or become imbalanced. Over the course of the entire research project, in thirty-nine sessions in the exoskeleton, Thibault covered only 145 meters in a cumulative total of 480 steps.

Exponentially more computing power will be needed if actual bipedal locomotion untethered from the supportive ceiling track is to be achieved, in addition to a more compact energy source. We are many iterations and vast financial expenditure away from this ungainly technology being anything that could be used to walk around a home or public place. As the authors of the published paper point out, however, the primary aim of the project was not to create a working exoskeleton or even facilitate Thibault's walking. His walking was essentially a visually arresting and culturally resonant deployment of the core focus of the study, a sensitive but long-lasting neural implant.[58] Having crossed this threshold, Thibault is now practicing using his brain implants to drive a motorized wheelchair, almost the identical wheelchair he was capable of steering before his neurotransmitter was implanted, using the remaining capacity in his right upper arm. Practically speaking, Thibault may have had a fun adventure in science, but it is unlikely to make any significant difference for his mobility or independence in years to come.

A disproportionate number of those who become paralyzed through a spinal injury already do not have adequate healthcare, leading them after paralysis to fall in disproportionate numbers even further below the poverty line.[59] Even if sufficient basic healthcare for the most needy was to be available, this particular technological route will never be a viable solution to their paralysis and the mobility limitations that attend it. It is a technology invented by the wealthy, which, if ever made functional, will be used only by those with access to substantial wealth. Even if neural implants were developed for Thibault, the remarkable imbalance between the cost and invasive nature of their installation and the limited benefit they give him makes it clear that they are intended to benefit others and have already benefited Benabid and Clinatec. Given that research on ameliorating a wide range of disabilities very often goes unfunded and given the relatively small numbers of patients who will use it, all indicators point to experiments of this type being directed not really at the good of the community of those with disabilities but at the investors who are rooting for it to look persuasive to the public.

We have now surveyed the economic, moral, and cultural landscape in which it makes perfect sense for popular articles discussing brain–machine interfaces to begin invariably by mentioning that these techniques were first developed to help people with brain or spinal cord injuries. It is precisely the rude primitivity to date of brain–computer link technologies sensitive enough to allow quadriplegics to walk that has allowed us to see that the therapy-enhancement distinction might not be abstractly morally sustainable, but it nevertheless remains at the heart of the goal–masking demanded by modern economic and technological imperatives. Projects like Thibault's exoskeleton are the cultural mask for a more basic ethical gambit. Their essential function is to harness a widespread public desire to eliminate a specific disability as an occasion to create a technology that can be more widely deployed once it has been proved to work and to not have obvious downsides. A therapeutic usage is the gateway through which an economic hope—a survival hope widely shared by the politicians and citizens of developed nations—can be offered to citizens. Can we really afford to pass up the economic advantages that will inevitably accrue to those who master this new technology and deploy it more widely?

Making Themselves Useful: Theological Thoughts on Using the Disabled

A nearly universal consensus has emerged among disability theologians on two basic points. First, disabled lives should not be instrumentalized to achieve the aims of others. It is this claim that energized secular movements like the emptying of the asylums, and that took form in Christian theology as an internal critique of the long-standing Christian presumption that the role of disabled people in God's economy was to be recipients of charity. That critique insisted that being vulnerable or different should never position anyone as an all-time recipient of charity for the exercise of the majority's need to "do good works to the needy." One of the early impulses funding the rise of the academic discourse of disability theology was the felt need to work out what follows in the wake of such an affirmation. Every human gaze that looks on a disabled person and sees the money that can be made from treating them (or from loudly broadcasting that they have been treated) falls foul of this first affirmation.

Second, the wide variations of human bodily and mental forms and capacities should be understood as a constitutive aspect of the vulnerability intrinsic to being creatures. The human race is more diverse than we imagine, and this diversity is good and should be affirmed. We should never seek to eliminate the differences of form and capacity that will always be present in the human community. This is often called the "normate assumption." To reject the assumption that all bodies should be judged against some universal norm is not to reject all therapeutic interventions that alter the body. It is to insist that all such interventions aim explicitly to ameliorate the sickness and suffering of individuals. There is no single norm for the functional human body to which every human ought to be made to conform. All hopes to eliminate disability entirely fall foul of this theological affirmation.

Might the first point prompt Christians to commit to refusing to use disabled lives to further their own agendas? Modern people have in fact very often refused to make any such commitment. The bodies of stillborn disabled fetuses and anomalously configured children's bodies have been a mainstay on which the imposing edifice of modern medical and genetic science has been built.[60] Modern philosophy in both its early and late modern varieties has almost invariably ignored physical and mental impairments except as useful illustrations of humans lacking supposedly universal human mental or physical traits.[61] Modern economics has systematically positioned those with disabilities alongside children and old people as nonproductive drags on the economy rather than productive contributors.[62]

It is this latter logic that almost certainly shaped the appeal made to Thibault to consider enrolling in a neural implant research protocol. Whether explicitly stated or not, as a young man of prime working age, Thibault could not but be aware of the widespread assumption that the technological elimination of disabilities is widely considered desirable among the late-modern public. Nor would it have been easy for him to ignore the assumption that by offering his body as a test bed for a socially useful technological innovation, he might transcend the class of nonproductive citizens to which disabled people are largely relegated in the developed world. One can also easily imagine the appeal to someone recently paralyzed at the beginning of the prime of life of being the center of a multimillion-euro research protocol at a world-class technology research lab. And under and through it all would no doubt filter the highly seductive call of the constantly present cultural narrative, that given powerful enough technology, the lame can walk like the deaf have come to hear. It may even be that in agreeing to be the subject of this research, Thibault was trying to take control of his own treatment trajectory, which, remarkably, is often absent in the treatment regime to which most spinal cord patients are subjected.[63]

Having traced the widespread cultural anxieties about disability and disruptive technological change that percolate through developed societies helps us make sense of what is going on in the stepping out of Thibault onto the global stage wearing his mind-activated exoskeleton. Without the twinned anxiety about disability as well as the potentially ethically and socially problematic aspects of neural implants, we cannot make sense of his story with Clinatec and, through the global media, with us. His story forces us to examine our participation in culturally configured anxieties among modern humanity about how to relate to its limits, its finitude.

Here disability theology can help us understand the importance of making peace with our finitude.[64] But education alone cannot dispel the problem of modern anxiety about our finitude, suggests Stacy Simplican. "When we presume that we can dismantle our anxiety about disability with knowledge, we reassert the fantasyland of the cognitively ideal world: that we have control over our minds; that we can decide to choose the way we think; and that we can, on demand, recalibrate the way we feel. This fantasy disavows disability all over again, as it sustains the familiar and fantastic cognitively ideal self—always troublesome, always seductive."[65] I have drawn attention to a related but equally seductive dream, the dream of the ideal, upright, and mobile physical self, and the anxieties that typically attach to our fears of losing this state (at least for those of us who have never really contemplated life without bodily mobility).

Let me end where I might have begun. Anxiety about finitude is part of the human condition, one that ought not be waved away. There has been a tendency among modern Christian theology to overshadow this aspect of human existence by overemphasizing human anxiety about sin. But anxiety about sin and judgment for sin is intertwined with and rests on anxiety about finitude and bodily death. Thus, the case of Thibault brings us before the truth that the Christian life is a *manner* or *mode* of living out our finitude, of responding to our finitude. Sin is that form of life that lives out creaturely finitude as if it could be surmounted. Those people who believe in the resurrection of Jesus Christ from the dead, also called Christians, are people who live their mortal lives as those transformed, literally metamorphized by that hope. In 1 Corinthians 15, the apostle Paul presents a vision of the resurrected or spiritual body as definitional for all Christian hopes for transformation:

> 40 There are both heavenly bodies and earthly bodies, but the glory of the heavenly is one thing, and that of the earthly is another. 41 There is one glory of the sun, and another glory of the moon, and another glory of the stars; indeed, star differs from star in glory. 42 So it is with the resurrection of the dead. What is sown is perishable, what is raised is imperishable. 43 It is sown in dishonor, it is raised in glory. It is sown in weakness, it is raised in power. 44 It is sown a physical body, it is raised a spiritual body. If there is a physical body, there is also a spiritual body. 45 Thus it is written, "The first man, Adam, became a living being"; the last Adam became a life-giving spirit. (NRSV)

Christian life is bodily, like everyone else's, yet is also animated by Christ as the "life-giving spirit" in a manner that changes the manner and mode of that body's activity. Paul does not deny but rather emphasizes that in the creaturely world the metamorphosis of the body that is death is a universal reality. All creaturely bodies come and go, changing form as they do so, metamorphizing. But Christ desires that these changeable bodies be transformed, by being animated by the Spirit.

Christians are left with the question of how to live this hope that transforms in a world without this hope. Without knowledge of eternal life, one can only hope to escape death and the limitations of finitude that can only appear as tragedies. Those who live only in the first Adam cannot but project the form of their current lives onto an undifferentiated span of future time to come. The only transformation possible for the first Adam is Nietzsche's recovery of the ancient idea of freedom as eternally accepting one's life and choices. From the viewpoint of the second Adam, however, this is an attempt at human self-transformation, the victory of our wills over death, finitude, and vulnerability.

A different way of living our fleshliness is held out in the resurrecting life of Christ, a life that can only be received through dying and vulnerability from the hand of the victor over death. The resurrecting power of God offers an alternative form of freedom to human lives than the dreams of the transhumanist, of which exoskeletons for the paraplegic are a telling icon. The exoskeleton may simulate lost mobility in some respects, and this may someday be a relatively good thing for people with mobility limitations. These are good things that might, perhaps accidentally,[66] emerge from transhumanist dreams. These dreams themselves are only another sad iteration of human resistance to the repentance and gratitude that leads to more wholesale transformation of not only our material bodies but our relationships to one another. Exoskeletons may simulate mobility, even if they spring from lives that have little inkling of genuinely new life.

There is more, much more, to say about disability from a theological perspective, but we will say none of this well if we have not made this crucial first move, of at least aspiring to learn what it means to come to terms with the implications of being finite creatures. To be freed from the sinful desire to be like gods takes not education but a savior who can show us the way through anxiety about illness and paralysis and physical suffering because he too has traversed it. By God's grace, Jesus Christ not only was resurrected with a glorified body but also showed us what it looks like to faithfully traverse the life of the finite creature, even through Gethsemane and Calvary.

NOTES

1   "Brain-Controlled Exoskeleton Helps Paralysed Man Learn to Walk Again in Technological Breakthrough," ABC News Australia, October 4, 2019, https://www.abc.net.au/news/2019-10-04/paralysed-man-learns -to-walk-again-brain-controlled-exoskeleton/11575882.

2   Clare Wilson, "A Mind-Controlled Exoskeleton Helped a Man with Paralysis Walk Again," New Scientist, October 3, 2019, https://institutions.newscientist.com/article/2218863-a-mind-controlled-exoskeleton-helped-a-man-with-paralysis-walk-again/.

3   Catherine Thorbecke, "Quadriplegic Man Walks with an Exoskeleton He Controls with His Brain," ABC News USA, October 4, 2019, https://abcnews.go.com/Technology/quadriplegic-man-walks-exoskeleton-controls-brain/story?id=66060762.

4   "World Cup 2014: First Kick Made by Paralyzed Man with the Help of Mind-Controlled Robot," YouTube video, 1:31, posted by Rajamanickam Antonimuthu, June 13, 2014, https://www.youtube.com/watch?app=desktop&v=TcAvtglo9Jg&pli=1.

5   Anita van Mil, Henrietta Hopkins, and Suzannah Kinsella, From Our Brain to the World: Views on the Future of Neural Interfaces; A Public Dialogue Research Programme Conducted on Behalf of the Royal Society (London: Creating Connections, Hopkins Van Mil, July 2019), 11.

6   Kelly McCarthy, "After 7 Years in Wheelchair, Groom Walks Down Aisle on His Wedding Day," ABC News USA, April 27, 2018, https://goodmorningamerica.com/family/story/years-wheelchair-groom-walks-aisle-wedding-day-54775343.

7   Disability critiques of this story: Helena L. Martin, "Martyrs and Monsters of the Avengers: Christianity and Disability in the Marvel Cinematic Universe," Journal of Disability & Religion, 24, no. 4 (2020): 453–61.

8   Alim Louis Benabid et al., "An Exoskeleton Controlled by an Epidural Wireless Brain–Machine Interface in a Tetraplegic Patient: A Proof-of-Concept Demonstration," Lancet Neurology 18, no. 12 (2019): 1120, https://doi.org/10.1016/S1474-4422(19)30321-7; "Watch Paralympian Jennifer French Stand Again Thanks to Bionic Implants," YouTube Video, 7:03, posted by World Science Festival, August 28, 2014, https://www.youtube.com/watch?v=CZCLBiUAKgo.

9   See Michael Banner, "A Doctrine of Human Being," in The Doctrine of God and Theological Ethics, ed. Alan Torrance and Michael Banner (London: T&T Clark International, 2006), 146. See also Tim Ingold, "'To Human' Is a Verb," in Verbs, Bones, and Brains: Interdisciplinary Perspectives on Human Nature, ed. A. Fuentes and A. Visala (Notre Dame: University of Notre Dame Press, 2017), 71–87.

10   Brian Brock, "Seeing Through the Data Shadow: Living the Communion of the Saints in a Surveillance Society," Surveillance and Society 16, no. 4 (2018): 533–45.

11   The most sophisticated and up-to-date Christian argument for the unsustainability of the therapy-enhancement distinction is Gerald

P. McKenny, *Biotechnology, Human Nature and Christian Ethics* (Cambridge: Cambridge University Press, 2018).

12 Van Mil, Hopkins, and Kinsella, *From Our Brain*.

13 There is a long history of dispute about cochlear implants in the deaf community, which turns upon the advisability of such operations to partially restore hearing while fundamentally rejecting the culture deaf people have built up over many generations. Raylene Paludneviciene and Irene W. Leigh, eds., *Cochlear Implants: Evolving Perspectives* (Washington, D.C.: Gallaudet University Press, 2011). There is a fundamental incompatibility between the desire to be "proudly deaf" and implants. Discourses premised on the value of Deafness and Deaf culture typically have little positive to say about implants. H.–Dirksen L. Bauman and Joseph J. Murray, eds., *Deaf Gain: Raising the Stakes for Human Diversity* (Minneapolis: University of Minnesota Press, 2014). The feature film *The Sound of Metal* (Pacific Northwest Pictures, 2020) powerfully depicts the visceral experience of deaf communities to cochlear implants as a technology inflicting social and physical violence on deaf communities.

14 Van Mil, Hopkins, and Kinsella, *From Our Brain*, 12.

15 Van Mil, Hopkins, and Kinsella, *From Our Brain*, 37.

16 Van Mil, Hopkins, and Kinsella, *From Our Brain*, 37.

17 Van Mil, Hopkins, and Kinsella, *From Our Brain*, 40.

18 Van Mil, Hopkins, and Kinsella, *From Our Brain*, 25.

19 Van Mil, Hopkins, and Kinsella, *From Our Brain*, 22.

20 Van Mil, Hopkins, and Kinsella, *From Our Brain*, 38

21 Don Idhe, *Technology and the Lifeworld: From Garden to Earth* (Bloomington: Indiana University Press, 1990), 74–80.

22 Van Mil, Hopkins, and Kinsella, *From Our Brain*, 12–13.

23 Van Mil, Hopkins, and Kinsella, *From Our Brain*, 13.

24 Van Mil, Hopkins, and Kinsella, *From Our Brain*, 64. Note that throughout the document no awareness is shown of the difference between the labels "Deaf people" and "deaf people." The quotation here offers a popular restatement uncannily reminiscent of the main thesis of Hans Reinders' now twenty–year–old book, *The Future of the Disabled in Liberal Society* (Notre Dame: University of Notre Dame Press, 2000).

25 The title of a recent and influential Rand report is telling: Marissa Norris and Alyson Youngblood, "Brain-Computer Interfaces Are Coming: Will We Be Ready?" Rand Corporation, August 27, 2020, https://www.rand.org/blog/articles/2020/08/brain-computer-interfaces-are-coming-will-we-be-ready.html.

26   Adam Greenfield, *Radical Technologies: The Design of Everyday Life* (London: Verso, 2018), chaps. 1–2.

27   Shoshana Zuboff outlines why we cannot participate in the wired society without surrendering data, and why the ubiquitous "terms of agreement" that we sign on an almost daily basis do not, and cannot, function in the way pre-internet contracts once worked. In terms of the pre-internet definition of the contract, they are best labelled "uncontracts." There is no "opt out" of data sharing in the wired world, only cosmetic increments of how much data we share. In this respect, the sociological fact that vanishingly few of us read the contracts that we sign online is in fact a tacit recognition that if we choose to opt out of data sharing, we will lose the functionality of the device or app that we are using. Zuboff, *The Age of Surveillance Capitalism: The Fight for the Future at the New Frontier of Power* (London: Profile Books, 2019), chs. 5–7.

28   The Hollywood blockbuster *Minority Report* (DreamWorks, 2002) first and most influentially announced the inevitability—but also the worrying implications—of the prediction-based politics of the "smart city."

29   The much-criticized policing approaches going under the labels "broken windows," "stop and search," "zero-tolerance," and "quality of life policing" are all dependent on surveillance technologies that can predict hot spots where extra policing—or especially heavy-handed policing—is believed to be effectively deployed. The intent to track the real-time location of the desire to menace or be antisocial is the policing analogue to the real-time location of consumer desire that is the engine of the click-and-buy economy. See Matt Taibbi, *I Can't Breathe: A Killing on Bay Street* (New York: Spiegel & Grau, 2017), 51–70.

30   Zuboff, *Age*, ch. 5

31   Zuboff, *Age*, 203 (emphasis original).

32   Zuboff, *Age*, 287.

33   Zuboff, *Age*, 289.

34   Danielle Carr, "Shit for Brains," *Baffler*, September 29, 2020, https://thebaffler.com/latest/shit-for-brains-carr.

35   "Robotic Exoskeleton Helps Paralyzed Man Race Marathons," YouTube video, 6:50, posted by "Freethink," August 7, 2019, https://www.youtube.com/watch?v=vBtXHGEezJA.

36   "Robotic Exoskeleton," YouTube video posted by "Freethink."

37   "iHuman Perspective: Neural Interfaces," Royal Society, September 10, 2019, https://royalsociety.org/topics-policy/projects/ihuman-perspective/.

38   In 2014 Benabid won a big-tech-sponsored prize for other neural interfacing projects. In a press release on the Clinatec website, his

links to big tech are front and center as well as the role of the media in sustaining the narrative I have described in this chapter. "Clinatec Chairman Alim-Louis Benabid Wins Breakthrough Prize," Clinatec, November 12, 2014, https://www.clinatec.fr/en/breakthrough-prize-2/.

> "Professor Benabid personifies the expertise and dedication that lead to new treatments for neurodegenerative diseases, disabilities, and cancer, which are at the center of Clinatec's research and development," said Jean Therme, director of technical research at CEA, the French alternative energies and atomic energy research institute that helped launch Clinatec. "The Breakthrough Prize and his many other awards offer encouragement to scientists and physicians at Clinatec and elsewhere who are dedicating their careers to improving the lives of patients."
>
> The Breakthrough Prize in Life Sciences Foundation, which also recognizes exceptional work in fundamental physics and mathematics, is sponsored by some of the world's biggest high-tech names. Founders include Sergey Brin, co-founder of Google; Anne Wojcicki, co-founder of the genetics company 23andMe; Alibaba CEO Jack Ma and his wife, Cathy Zhang; the Russian venture capitalist Yuri Milner and his wife, Julia Milner, and Facebook CEO Mark Zuckerberg and his wife, Priscilla Chan.
>
> The Breakthrough Prize in Life Sciences award was presented to Benabid and the other winners on Nov. 9 in Silicon Valley, Calif. The award ceremony will be televised in the U.S. as a simulcast on Discovery Channel and Science Channel on Nov. 15 and globally the weekend of Nov. 22 on BBC World News.

39   "Brain-Controlled Exoskeleton," ABC News Australia.

40   "Until medical experimentation is seen as an opportunity—and perhaps even an obligation—for everyone, I find it hard to justify the continued use of prisoners and the poor as experimental subjects." Stanley Hauerwas, *Suffering Presence: Theological Reflections on Medicine, the Mentally Handicapped and the Church* (Edinburgh: T&T Clark, 1986), 120.

41   Tim Denison, "Neural Interface Technologies: Industrial Perspectives," iHuman Working Group Paper, Royal Society, 2019, 4, https://royalsociety.org/-/media/policy/projects/ihuman/7-industry-perspectives.pdf?la=en-GB&hash=496F7DD87D39C979293CC5A568120D8A.

42   Denison, "Neural," 5.

43   Musk's Neuralink project has, however, been dogged by accusations of animal cruelty. Theo Wayt, "Elon Musk's Neuralink Allegedly Subjected Monkeys to 'Extreme Suffering,'" *New York Post*, February 10, 2022.

44 Rebecca Heilweil, "Elon Musk Is One Step Closer to Connecting a Computer to Your Brain," *Vox*, August 28, 2020, https://www.vox.com/recode/2020/8/28/21404802/elon-musk-neuralink-brain-machine-interface-research.

45 On May 7, 2021, Musk publicly announced on *Saturday Night Live* that he has been diagnosed with Asperger's syndrome, positioning that announcement as an explanation for some of his more well-known social infractions. The announcement raises a host of questions, not least why Musk is using a diagnostic label that has been officially retired by the medical profession, and whether it is even possible to debate his right to identify as he would like. Adam McCrimmon, "What Happened to Asperger's Syndrome?" *Conversation*, March 8, 2018, http://theconversation.com/what-happened-to-aspergers-syndrome-89836; Victoria McGeer, "The Thought and Talk of Individuals with Autism: Reflections on Ian Hacking," *Metaphilosophy* 40, nos. 3–4 (2009): 517–30.

46 Carr, "Shit for Brains" (emphasis original).

47 Carr, "Shit for Brains."

48 Alexandre Gonfalonieri, "What Brain-Computer Interfaces Could Mean for the Future of Work," *Harvard Business Review*, October 6, 2020, https://hbr.org/2020/10/what-brain-computer-interfaces-could-mean-for-the-future-of-work.

49 Liam Stoker, "Military Exoskeletons Uncovered: Ironman Suits a Concrete Possibility," Army Technology, June 11, 2020, accessed May 13, 2021, https://www.army-technology.com/features/featuremilitary-exoskeletons-uncovered-ironman-suits-a-concrete-possibility/.

50 Gonfalonieri, "Brain-Computer."

51 P. W. Singer, *Wired for War: The Robotics Revolution and Conflict in the 21st Century* (New York: Penguin, 2009), 71–74.

52 "How Exoskeletons Can Help People With Paraplegia Walk Again," Spinal Cord Injury Zone, February 15, 2021, https://spinalcordinjuryzone.com/news/54908/how-exoskeletons-can-help-people-with-paraplegia-walk-again.

53 Stacy Clifford Simplican, *The Capacity Contract: Intellectual Disability and the Question of Citizenship* (Minneapolis: University of Minnesota Press, 2015), 57.

54 Gareth M. Thomas, *Down Syndrome Screening and Reproductive Politics: Care, Choice, and Disability in the Prenatal Clinic* (Abingdon, U.K.: Routledge, 2017); David Patterson and Alberto C. S. Costa, "History of Genetic Disease: Down Syndrome and Genetics—A Case of Linked Histories," *Nature Reviews Genetics* 6 (2005): 137–47.

55 "Deep Brain Stimulation," American Association of Neurological Sur-geons, https://www.aans.org/en/Patients/Neurosurgical-Conditions-and-Treatments/Deep-Brain-Stimulation.

56 Martin Sullivan, "Subjected Bodies: Paraplegia, Rehabilitation, and the Politics of Movement," in *Foucault and the Government of Disability*, rev. ed., ed. Shelley Tremain (Ann Arbor: University of Michigan Press, 2015), 27–44.

57 Benabid et al., "Exoskeleton."

58 "This study describes the first successful long-term use of wireless epidural multi-channel recorders that were bilaterally implanted in a patient with tetraplegia. . . . All the technical elements that are required for long-term human clinical application (epidural recording, wireless power and emission, online decoding of many ECoG chan-nels, and being totally embedded) have been combined for the first time." Benabid et al., "Exoskeleton," 1120.

59 Roni Caryn Rabin, "Study Raises Estimate of Paralyzed Americans," *New York Times*, April 20, 2009, https://www.nytimes.com/2009/04/21/health/21para.html.

60 Armand Marie Leroi, *Mutants: On the Form, Varieties and Errors of the Human Body* (London: Harper Perennial, 2005).

61 Licia Carlson, *The Faces of Intellectual Disability: Philosophical Reflec-tions* (Bloomington: Indiana University Press, 2010); Angela Woods, *The Sublime Object of Psychiatry: Schizophrenia in Clinical and Cultural Theory* (Oxford: Oxford University Press, 2011).

62 David T. Mitchell with Sharon L. Snyder, *The Biopolitics of Disability: Neoliberalism, Ablenationalism, and Peripheral Embodiment* (Ann Arbor: University of Michigan Press, 2015); Michael Oliver and Colin Barnes, *The New Politics of Disablement*, rev. ed. (Basingstoke, U.K.: Palgrave Macmillan, 2012), ch. 3; Gary L. Albrecht, *The Disability Business: Reha-bilitation in America* (Newbury Park, Calif.: Sage, 1992).

63 Sullivan, "Subjected Bodies," in Tremain, *Foucault*.

64 Deborah Beth Creamer, *Disability and Christian Theology: Embodied Lim-its and Constructive Possibilities* (Oxford: Oxford University Press, 2009).

65 Simplican, *Capacity Contract*, 92

66 Most effects of technology are unanticipated. Don Idhe, "The Designer Fallacy and Technological Imagination," in *Ironic Technics* (Copenhagen: Automatic Press / VIP, 2008), 19–30; Andrew Pickering, *The Mangle of Practice: Time Agency & Science* (Chicago: University of Chicago Press, 1995); Bruno Latour, *Aramis, or The Love of Technology*, trans. Catherine Porter (Cambridge, Mass.: Harvard University Press, 1996).

8

CHRISTIAN TRANSHUMANISM IN CONTEXT

The Relevance of Race

Terri Laws

Transhumanism, as a matter within the field of bioethics, largely overlooks race as a contextual topic. In a volume on Christian transhumanism, the field needs to make space for the context of race—on its own sociocultural terms. Contributors in this collection agreed to this philosophical grounding during our November 2019 gathering before the start of the American Academy of Religion annual meeting. In this essay, I focus on two of the group statements that emerged during the meeting, as they related to my communities of concern and research. The two group statements that influenced this essay are: (1) "All theology is contextual. As such, vulnerable bodies are also contextual. So, theology and guiding practices related to them must be broad frameworks that foster inclusiveness." And (2) "Christians should uphold their responsibility of caring for the marginalized, and those hindered by 'biological limitations' who experience biological and social limitations (sickness, disease, and suffering) because of the inevitable lack of access to bioenhancement technologies within the lag time of equitable access for all."[1] Race is a context that is largely missing from transhumanist discourse. In this essay, I argue that acceptance of these philosophical statements applied to the inclusion of race and ethnicity in Christian transhumanism begins with an empathetic stance—in its content, topics, and movement. The aim of approaches to context and inclusion that begin in empathy should seek to transform the legacy of rational distrust borne out of the power and authority given to racism from both scientific medicine and Christianity as culturally devised in colonial British North America. I begin with a brief history of how the Christian project in colonial British North America developed out of an exploitative rather than empathetic stance. I present this same failure of an empathetic stance from scientific medicine. Next, I present three approaches to an empathetic stance for inclusion in the development of Christian transhumanism. Finally, I offer a case study of how an empathetic approach achieves both a racially inclusive expansion of bioenhancement technologies and the Christian transhumanist movement, in general.

AFRICAN AMERICAN RELIGION AS A CONTEXTUAL EXAMPLE

Scholars from two academic fields associated with transhumanist discourse relevant to this volume (religious studies and bioethics) have proclaimed that their fields have a race problem. Prior to the declarations for context by the contributors to this volume, Catherine Myser argued that there is a presumed and embedded "white normativity" in bioethics that "risk[s] reproducing white privilege and white supremacy in its theory, method, and practices."[2] Laura McTighe wrote her claim directly: "Religious Studies has a race problem."[3] The field of Black[4] religious studies examines the problem and processes of race, argues that its existence has serious consequences, and proposes ways that the problems can be corrected through expanded Black religious symbols, collective agency, and changed behaviors by perpetrators of injustice. More recently, there has been a growth in whiteness studies within religion.

As a religious research and social problem, as it is addressed in this essay, race is an arbitrary category made consequential through various forms or systems of racism that point to disparate, negative experiences in the daily and generational lives of Black Americans. Race remains a relevant category for discourse because of experiences and practices of racism as a power dynamic. Experiences of racism are descriptive and empirical. Practices of racism are dispersed through social, cultural, and political narratives and are frequently disputed, trivialized, and marginalized. The existence of racism requires ongoing contextual interpretation through intellectual and pragmatic address. Religion—as defined by religious institutions, divisive teachings, activities and authority figures and the research methods of scientific medicine—are both implicated in the "invention" of race and the spread of the detriments of racism and exclusion. Unfortunately, the transhumanist movement and its faith-based counterpart give little attention to race. For Christian transhumanism to minimize taking these intellectual habits and practices into the future, it must, first, study the history of race and racism in Christianity and, second, choose to develop and/or accept inclusive contextual approaches as its movement and conceptual frames emerge. My focus here is the African American case.

Sociologist of religion Robert P. Jones is a scholar who has turned his search for understanding to the study of white Christianity. Jones recalls his Baptist and Methodist upbringing in the U.S. South as demonstrating a powerful, caring, and cohesive religious community. He notes, however, that he "didn't learn much about how [his] religious tradition, which had undeniably done so much good for so many people, including [himself], had also been simultaneously entangled in justifying unspeakable racial violence, bigotry, and ongoing indifference to African Americans' claims to equality and justice."[5] Jones writes compellingly about white Christians' connections to historical episodes of white supremacy, such as biblical myths deployed to justify the dehumanizing institution of the race-based enslavement of Africans in colonial British North America and ritual, vigilante, anti-Black lynching held in a family picnic atmosphere, often after Sunday worship services.[6] These horrific cruelties stand in stark contrast against persons who claim the same faith tradition. Jones focuses in on the differential deployment of race among Christian leaders, including the 1963 Birmingham, Alabama, Civil Rights Campaign and the famous "Letter from Birmingham City Jail" written by Reverend Dr. Martin Luther King Jr. in response to local white pastors.[7]

In the letter, King morally indicts these white church leaders. As the Easter season neared, King was in jail in Birmingham for conducting nonviolent civil rights protests that he, other Black ministers, and Black citizens led in the city. From his cell, he read an open letter written by local white pastors and published in a local newspaper in January 1963. King expressed disappointment at the interpretation of Christianity that the white leaders chose to represent. According to Washington, the writers had been "eight prominent 'liberal' Alabama clergymen, all white."[8] These pastors believed that the battle for civil rights should remain in the courts rather than in the streets—without the direct-action tactics that King and his lieutenants so skillfully used.[9] In their open letter, the white pastors chose to attempt to redirect the actions of King and the protesters. Instead, the clergymen could have sided with the just cause of the protesters in the fight for equal humanity by providing instruction on Christian justice to white city leaders, who were their congregants, and who were withholding the benefits of citizenship from Black Birmingham residents. Whites and Blacks may have shared the same faith tradition in name, but, as King observed in a 1960 *Meet the Press* interview, "11:00 a.m. on Sundays is the most segregated or one of the most segregated hours in the week."[10] Their differing interpretations of their shared faith was based on their contexts. In general, too often, Christianity in the U.S. context has been unwilling to acknowledge that it has a history *and* continuing legacy of viewing (and, charitably, misunderstanding) Black people through a dehumanized or lesser-than lens. Ironically, many Black people have historically chosen to understand their faith as a means of correcting this perspective by reading Christianity through a (group) self-affirming lens.

Philip Butler observes that there is scant analysis of the effects on or of ideas and experiences of race and ethnicity within the transhumanist movement.[11] As Butler reads transhumanism, the category of race is "inconsequential"[12] in the way that sociology discusses it as a marker of epistemological, social, cultural, and institutional experience and as a legacy of enslavement. Instead, race refers to the human race. For Butler, race and ethnicity are relevant as a continuation of Enlightenment thinkers' subjugation that living in the experience of Blackness makes those beings less than human, inferior to Europeans, especially northern Europeans. Butler arrives at three reasons why transhumanism has failed to construct an address to race and ethnicity: "a lack of connection to these events; a lack of empathy with those who suffered under its proceedings; and a lack of experience exploring the weight or the depth of the histories, bodies, and lineages connected to race, ethnicity, and power."[13] Any one or all of these three lines of reason related to the failure of transhumanism to adequately engage race can be true in the African American case. Even more importantly, each line provides evidence to demonstrate why understanding this history of engagement (or, in this case, the lack thereof) with Black folk, Black ideas, and Black experience is not a past intellectual exercise. Rather, its ongoing negative assumptions, though more subtle than in fifteenth-century science and seventeenth-century Christian theology, require diligence to avoid being passed along in the epistemologies, ethics, and procedural acts of the twenty-first-century Christian transhumanist movement. Direct address, like the nonviolent direct action of the late twentieth-century civil rights movement, helps to unravel the misguided narrative in transhumanist discourse that race is inconsequential. The history of religion is integral to the raced experience, and contemporary health inequity scholarship offers empirical evidence of differential experience that is not erased by social class (think Black maternal death rates). How, then, can movement scholars and advocates avoid race and ethnicity becoming a negative part of the construction of Christian transhumanism by giving attention to their context?

An empathetic contextual approach to Christian transhumanism must be willing to directly risk engagement with race in the same way as the faith-influenced direct-action protesters. To do so presents a chicken-and-egg dilemma: Does construction of an empathetic contextual perspective in the Christian transhumanism movement begin with the expansion of a theological category? Or do we approach this contextual understanding by developing a question from the human experience of bioenhancement to be answered with a theological response? Is either beginning sufficient?

Approaches to the Construction of Contextual Transhumanist Theology

If past is prologue, the history of humanity's treatment of peoples different from themselves offers a guide to what to look for in the present and the future development of Christian transhumanism. The first task, the decision that human difference is important, was agreed to in principle by contributors in this volume even as many secular transhumanists argue that this type of race categorization is a nonissue in the examination of biotechnologies and the development of transhumanist discourse. For a Christian transhumanist, moral obligation is embedded within the foundations of the faith tradition. Tested by the religious scholars of his day, Jesus demonstrates the continuity between himself and Judaic law. He simplifies the ancient and contemporary teachings to two key aspects of theology: relationship with God and relationship with other humans.[14] In Luke's version of the scene, it is followed by the parable of the good Samaritan. Among the multiple lessons therein is the teaching about cross-cultural empathy. Spoken by Jesus himself, the ethic is to love and respect humanity through the dictum of "love thy neighbor as thyself." Justice is said to be what love looks like in public.[15] The capacity to love, the capacity to seek justice, is forged in empathy. Both of these have complex meanings, but the commandment to love cannot be fulfilled without first identifying, somehow, with the object of that love—empathizing with them.[16] The question is, how shall Christian transhumanism willfully infuse its technologies and discourse with empathy? As an example, the lack of empathy for Black women is producing a growing body of literature crossing theology, ethics, history, and the social sciences, with constructive proposals—through a variety of genre—which provides helpful fodder to develop contextual transhumanism.

Empathetic Embrace as a Methodological Approach to Contextual Recognition

In her literary and cultural research on the content and intellectual development of difference, Esther Jones argues for the need to reinfuse medicine with empathy and compassion, characteristics, she asserts, that have declined as science within medicine has expanded its influence on ideas about human difference and widened the distance between people in other people groups. Deirdre Cooper Owens provides an examination of this troublesome loss of affect in reproductive care as it moved from the female-dominated midwifery to the mid-nineteenth-century development of the male-dominated field of gynecology, which was advanced by scientific activity including experimentation and case narratives in medical journals.[17] "Medicine—whether as a system, institution, or discourse—wields, quite arguably, the most power in our contemporary era to identify, name, and categorize difference. In spite of its humanistic and altruistic underpinnings, those who embody difference are treated differentially within the medical establishment."[18] As a matter of difference, Owens' argument continues, the application of science in medicine has been especially focused in the pathologizing and exploitation of Black bodies and women's bodies, specifically in sexualized ways.[19] As medicine and science are connected to transhumanism, this past is not inconsequential on racial or gender cases, and cannot be so easily dismissed. To demonstrate her point, Jones points to biographical episodes about J. Marion Sims and Georges Cuvier.[20] As physician–scientists they contributed to what today is interpreted as historical experiences of medicalized trauma. In the interest of space, I will detail only the matter of Sims.

In recent years, increasingly, members of the general public have become familiar with Sims' name and fame: he is credited with the mid–nineteenth-century development of surgical treatment of vesicovaginal fistula repairs, primarily created during lengthy childbirth, and the development of the speculum for use during vaginal medical examination.[21] This type of fistula caused extreme incontinence and an odorous presence resulting in social isolation besides its biological issues. Three enslaved Black women are named in many historical accounts as the objects of Sims' experimentation. In his memoir, the doctor acknowledges "three to four more,"[22] and other accounts identify that as many as eleven enslaved women are believed to have been operated upon.[23] The named three—Betsey, Lucy, and Anarcha—bore multiple, painful experimental surgeries that eventually earned Sims the title of the "father of gynecology." Late-twentieth–century readers critique Sims as racist and sexist for operating on the enslaved women without anesthesia in his efforts to perfect his instruments and surgical repair technique. In 2018, advocates accomplished relocation of a Sims statue from New York City's Central Park;[24] Sims' portrait was removed from the University of Alabama; and the American Urogynecologic Society ceased the use of his name from a prestigious annual lecture.[25]

As a matter of ethical reasoning, it is considered, by some, to be ethically anachronistic to critique an ethical stance taken during an earlier period through the lens of a different, especially contemporary ethical understanding. That is, it is inappropriate to evaluate a historical ethical episode by a later or contemporary ethical standard. In common language: times change. In the case of Sims, contemporary critics such as the activists whose protests resulted in the removal of Sims' memorials refer to him as sexist and racist, in part, because of his lack of the use of anesthesia. Today, it is considered caring and empathetic medicine to anticipate the need to relieve pain during surgery, and unethical to fail to plan for post-surgical pain, or worse, to refuse to address the need for pain relief. Owens notes that the use of anesthesia during Sims' day was more common in dentistry than surgery; the approach to surgery was to work quickly.[26] Accordingly, Sims would have relied on quickly completing the women's operations so each patient would not bleed profusely, endangering her life. That said, Owens is not arguing that Sims' actions were meritorious and without criticism; she is providing additional contemporaneous technological context. On the other hand, L. Lewis Wall, a physician and philosopher, thinks Sims has been misjudged.[27] Wall asserts an empathetic understanding of the value gained from Sims' experimental surgeries. His interpretation that Anarcha gave consent overlooks that it was Sims who says that Anarcha gave her consent, yet there is no evidence of her direct voice. Furthermore, by Wall's own selection of facts from Sims' memoir, Anarcha "underwent 30 operations before Sims was able to close the holes in her bladder and rectum."[28] He accuses "some modern writers [of having] denounced Sims with the kind of righteous indignation that is usually heard only from pulpits."[29] Wall believes that the focus in the Sims historical account ought to be on medical discovery—the science—the very set of practices, we are reminded, that Esther Jones argued have reduced empathy in medicine, and that Owens asserted that when applied within the context of medicine and difference had the power to exploit the bodies of Black women, in particular. This is certainly suggested in Wall's interpretation of the valuing of the scientific gains without regard for devaluing the dynamics of Anarcha's subjectivity.

Ethically and culturally to merely reify the science is too narrow; it misses the importance of context. Sims acknowledges that his community (and he, himself) initially understood him primarily as a family practitioner. As such, he was called upon to treat illnesses among local whites and their Black slaves; this is also key contextual information. In Sims' retelling, he highlights his initial disinterest in attempting to address the severe incontinence (and the accompanying odors and social displacement) caused by issues such as torn bladders. (He describes one woman as having developed the fistula during an excruciating seventy-two-hour labor.) Sims was made aware of multiple cases. Only after a local white woman developed a similar type of fistula after being thrown from a pony did he choose to do more than take note that she was in agony.[30] Before the latter case, he saw the fistula issue for the enslaved women as an interesting "surgical curiosity" yet an incurable condition.[31] There is additional context through which Sims' experiments should be understood for its ethics and its empathetic content. With the end of the legal importation of Africans for enslavement, the American institution depended on in-country slavery to be sustained and grow. Black women were used as "breeders."[32] This growth was achieved through changes in legal structures as early as the seventeenth century. Laws were revised to have the status of a child follow the status of the mother. Previously, the legal status of a child followed that of the father. In other words, after the change, if a mother was a slave, so, too, would the newborn be, even if the father was a free man, Black or white.[33] Each child that an enslaved woman bore added property and wealth for the owners of the enslaved woman. This was "reproductive labor."[34] Thus, the value of these Black women was in their labor, whether that was working in the field, domestic work, or breeding children.

A belief that enslaved women encumbered within such interlocking systems could give unfettered consent is dismissive of the power and economic dynamics embedded in the doctor's memoir. Sims proposed the use of the enslaved women for his surgical experiments, promising not to "endanger their lives"; in exchange, he would pay their owners for their keep except for taxes and the women's clothing needs.[35] Sims wanted to assure the local slaveholders that he would not harm their property, the enslaved women in whose medical issue he previously had little interest but now saw as a technological opportunity. The fullness of this context must be considered to understand the relevance of reinserting empathy and to be able to recognize the context in its contemporary manifestations that devalue Black women even in their vulnerable state as patients. This is the type of lack of empathy that plagues Black women in the clinical setting when disproportionately their voices are not acknowledged[36] and when medical professionals believe that Black people, in general, are less prone to feel pain.[37] Recall that Esther Jones' research question is whether narrative medicine achieves its aim to humanize scientific medicine by reinserting empathy.

Concluding that the efforts and techniques of narrative medicine insufficiently meet the challenge to reinsert empathy into scientific medicine, Jones proposes instead to study Black woman-authored science fiction. These stories help to deconstruct the link to the bodies that scientific medicine has pathologized, which used science to construct racial and gender hierarchies and then to rank Black women low on those scales.[38] Jones analyzes three books from Black women–authored science fiction. In them, she notes characteristics that overlap between the works and real life. Minoritized protagonists are Black women or girls who serve a spiritual as well as a healing purpose in the stories. Illnesses in their individual lives represent social or societal ills in need of healing. Jones observes that, in two of the three stories (*Who Fears Death* and Octavia Butler's *Parable of the Sower* and *Parable of the Talents*), "narrative authority is represented by controlling documents that inculcate widespread problematic beliefs and practices. How these controlling narratives operate in the world is a fundamental issue, and the protagonists engage in rewriting of such narratives as a starting point for devising a new ethics of relationality."[39] Religio-spirituality and relationality are central to the protagonists and to understanding the disorder and healing in these stories. The process that Jones explains as occurring within these works can be applied as a method to heal contextual, Christian transhumanism before it develops with disorder. The use of contextual sources—in their own voices—is what contextual religious studies has offered to every other branch of religious scholarship. Why not, also, to transhumanism?

Empathetic Embrace as a Discursive Centric Approach

For the next treatment of empathy as an approach to infusing contextual address, I turn to Philip Butler, who I cited above as identifying empathy as a possible reason that race-as-difference is largely missing from the transhumanism movement. He argues for a Black transhuman liberation theology. He credits Michael Shapiro as being one of the few transhumanist scholars who acknowledges race. However, in doing so, according to Butler, Shapiro finds "race and ethnicity [to be] 'problematic classifications'" and that such categories "must not persist."[40] Categories such as race and ethnicity highlight the "divide in access to, or reception of, newer technologies."[41]

Butler proposes that "for [a category such as] Blackness to be maintained . . . Black folks [would need to] shed our humanity."[42] The continuance of a category such as race will make its already existing access and adoption disparities worse. Butler agrees with Shapiro's assessment about disparities but finds Shapiro's alternative—to choose to eliminate race as a category in order to accommodate this problem with access and adoption—to be unimaginable and untenable. This is especially salient to thinkers such as Butler (and the author of this chapter), for whom race is central to his identity and his very being. The elimination suggestion fails in the expression of empathy; it also misses the relevance of producing bioenhancement for the needs of diverse groups. Instead, he posits Black liberation theology as the starting place to envision a contextual approach to Black participation in the transhumanist movement. Butler constructs his framing around neuroscience for his hermeneutical application. This contextual approach engages a bioenhancement topic alongside a key contribution of Black theology to the academic study of religion. James Cone's[43] Black theology became relevant and helped to develop a new field because it spoke to its transitioning sociocultural times, engaging the theologies and philosophies represented by Martin Luther King and Malcolm X, nonviolence and Black Power. Its vital theological construction, Cone argued, was that in such a moment Jesus would be in the midst of that which was troublesome. Jesus would not shy away from the problem of finding a way to include Blackness; rather, he would identify as Black with all of the challenges that it brings. To be clear, explaining Cone is not the focus of Butler's text. He offers much more by posing a Black transhuman liberation theological argument, but, for this essay, this initial point must be understood to argue for why context still matters in the development of Christian transhumanism. Cone's contribution to the idea of context cannot be overstated. Professional organizations such as the American Academy of Religion, the Society for Biblical Literature, and American Society for Bioethics and the Humanities all now include contextually focused affinity groups and presentations. Cone's construction did not begin in the study of an abstract God, as his theological training had taught him. Rather his Black theology spoke to God's power to rectify the oppression of racism, a major social and existential issue of concern to Black people, which Cone proposed to solve through religious constructions. The construction was based on daily concerns of history and contemporary experience rather than from the speculative, abstract vantage point of God.

This idea of addressing daily, practical concerns is where a contextual approach to Christian transhumanism lies within the African cultural tradition of "both/and" reasoning where there is no hard line between characteristics that may appear to be oppositional. Think, for example, about the relationship between the sacred and the secular where there is no hard binary that separates the two. In music, the blues, a Black cultural form, is closely related to gospel music, and soul singers such as Sam Cooke and Aretha Franklin crossed over from singing in church to concert halls. More recently, *American Idol* winner Fantasia often invokes the faith of her grandmother and inserts gospel numbers during her pop music concerts.

Like Jones and Butler—each in their separate projects—I see empathy as vital to the Christian transhumanist movement race discourse. Butler noted the *lack* of empathy as one of the potential reasons why the transhumanist movement does not engage race. Jones wants to reclaim empathy in the space that science is taking up within medicine. I agree with these authors, and my interest in empathy is as an element of human flourishing—well-being, a life worth living.[44] My "both/and" proposal calls for empathy and for a contextual approach that centers bioenhancements specifically relevant to African Americans. Such an approach focuses on health disparities that cause greater suffering and death.

Empathetic Embrace as Response to Contextual Experience:
A "Both/And" Approach

The embrace—demand, even—is for the centrality of empathy as a religious ideal with intentional functionality and activity, not merely ideas. Its inclusion is supported within basic principles of Christian theology—to love God with all one's heart and mind and to love one's neighbor as one loves oneself—and, I would argue, that to be considered empathetic, it must be contextual to the receiving party. As a cultural form, Black religion is structurally pragmatic. In this sense, it follows its complex African roots spread around the globe through the African Traditional Religion (ATR) that the Africans brought with them during the trans-Atlantic slave trade. ATR was grounded by a Supreme God, other minor deities or spiritual beings who met the local needs for daily living, as well as revered ancestors who guided them through life by imparting wisdom. In the African American contextual approach, then, bioenhancement should be centered in an empathetic impulse that fits its religio-pragmatic wisdom of caring, with the purpose of healing, and that healing should be focused on eliminating the suffering in health disparity and inequity. The parable of the good Samaritan is named for the one who has been identified as the primary actor, yet his activity met the need of the one who was injured. This is not merely a good deed; it is a contextual response. I should note that—applied to African Americans (and other marginalized communities), who are too little a part of the transhumanism discourse (because inclusion takes considerable effort)—I am *not* insinuating that marginalized communities are victims without agency. Rather, the good Samaritan story is relevant because of its demonstration of met need in accordance with the one who has been harmed—a feature of "the least of these" theology, fully empathetic. Transhumanism has the opportunity to intentionally target Black life for what it needs, thereby meeting the contextual approach in the empathetic criterion and the relief of somatic suffering. The story of Victoria Gray is an example.

Victoria Gray is a thirty-six-year-old Mississippi mother who experienced her first sickle cell crisis at the age of three months.[45] Sickle cell disease presents as misshapen red blood cells. A regular red blood cell is oval-shaped and flexible enough to move through blood vessels. However, with sickle cell disease, red blood cells are shaped like crescents with pointed ends, and they are less flexible.[46] Essentially, they can become stuck in blood vessels, cutting off the vital flow of blood to the rest of the body or to an organ on the other side of the sickle cell. A crisis incident is one of these episodes; it can be extremely painful and damage vital organs. Imagine a three-month-old infant,[47] unable to communicate her pain sensation other than through crying. Then imagine living with the possibility of the unpredictable return of a crisis episode for more than thirty years. Gray has reported that an ordinary task such as doing the laundry could take the mother of four more than a single day to complete because she did not have sufficient energy. In the United States, this disease disproportionately affects African Americans. Periodically, the medical establishment (research and clinical) has given attention to this painful suffering and life-limiting condition. In 2018, sickle cell disease, cancer, and blindness became CRISPR gene-therapy research candidates. National Public Radio (NPR) was granted exclusive access to follow Gray's story of participation in experimental medicine for hopeful clinical improvement.[48] She entered a sickle cell gene-editing trial in Nashville, and NPR periodically reports on her progress. Gray's story is relevant to this discussion of contextual Christian transhumanism on multiple levels.

Allowing for CRISPR technology as a form of bioenhancement, its use to edit the mutated gene that causes Gray's (and other patients') sickle cell disease can contribute to healing her future health as well as to offer a step toward revising the exploitative narrative at the center of the history of African Americans, medicine, and religion. Although the NPR reporting does not examine an empathetic motivation that guides the research team that recruited Gray, her self-reported improvement in the quality of her daily life is itself a measure of the empathetic value of sickle cell gene editing. Two years out, Gray continues to be closely monitored. During the COVID-19 pandemic, she had energy to join mothers from across the country who supplemented their children's virtual education. She has the hope of being able to be present for her children's graduations and weddings, or just to jump on their backyard trampoline. This is the individual-level effect. Specific sustained attention to technologies that intentionally address health disparities that disproportionately affect African Americans and offer improvement for its inherent value in their lives is actually somewhat rare.[49] For example, historical experimental medicine to improve the stamina of enslaved Black people was not for the inherent value to Blacks themselves;

it was for the value that it offered enslavers.[50] More often systemic improvements are intentionally colorblind so as not to appear to advantage any one group. This falsely conceals the different experiences by groups within the aggregate. To reveal these sorts of concealments is the point of context whether it is related to medicine or theology. The original, multisite study that Victoria Gray joined has filled its planned recruitment of forty-five patients. At the collective level, this is the sort of research that can go a long way toward healing Black distrust of medicine and the theology that willfully denigrated Black people in search of white supremacy. Victoria Gray credits her religious faith with giving her the capacity to take the risk to be the first sickle cell patient to volunteer for gene editing. Hopefully, the other forty-four patients will have as good results as she has experienced.

CONCLUSION

Black contextual theology emerged during the late 1960s, with the work of James Cone rising to notable prominence in the publication of *Black Theology and Black Power* followed by *A Black Theology of Liberation*. Other forms of contextual religious scholarship have followed in the ensuing decades. As a human experience, bioenhancement as one form of transhumanism should be no different. Moral bioenhancement can include regulating hate and developing empathy; the purpose of these would be to offer improvements from the group subjective perspective of the receiver, not the developer or movement leaders. Though this may be viewed as a challenge, how would the design of such bioenhancement be any different from other forms of theological hermeneutics? Thinkers who have contributed, and continue to contribute, to varying disciplines of contextual Christian scholarship (and faith) came from different sociological experiences. Sometimes these new approaches were welcomed as an opportunity to understand the expansiveness of the human condition. At other times they were seen as chipping away at the universal human experience and wholly unnecessary, if not heretical. But within those sociological groups there was also the possibility of being included in the Christian family in a way that matched lived experience. To better represent human flourishing in the bioenhancement world to come, these philosophical ideals and lessons learned from the entrance of contextual theology can and should be transferred to Christian contextual approaches to transhumanism. The Black freedom struggle continues to be religio–spiritually influenced. Research in Black American expressions of religion within healthcare—folk and biomedicine—also continues to locate a relationship of religio-spirituality, including decision–making on controversial topics such as medical aid in dying and inequities in the healthcare experience. Given the periodic acknowledgement of a race problem in its lacking presence in broad Christian scholarship, in medicine, and in the scholarship at their intersection in bioethics, race warrants direct address in transhumanism, with a particular moral obligation to do so within Christian transhumanism.

NOTES

1   Meeting group reference, November 19, 2019.

2   Catherine Myser, "Differences from Somewhere: The Normativity of Whiteness in Bioethics in the United States," *American Journal of Bioethics* 3, no. 2 (2003): 1–11.

3   Laura McTighe, "Roundtable: 'Religio–racial Identity' as Challenge and Critique, Introduction," *Journal of the American Academy of Religion* 88, no. 2 (2020): 299–303.

4   In this essay, I am using the terms "Black" and "African American" interchangeably in relation to the people group with cultural roots in Africa. However, it should be noted that not all Black Americans or other Black people are African Americans with a heritage of enslavement. For example, some Blacks may have a contemporary, self-determined immigrant experience.

5   Robert P. Jones, *White Too Long: The Legacy of White Supremacy in American Christianity* (New York: Simon & Schuster, 2020), 74.

6   Jones, *White Too Long*, 28–33.

7   Jones, *White Too Long*, 75.

8   James Melvin Washington, "Introductory Abstract to 'Letter from Birmingham City Jail,'" in *A Testament of Hope: The Essential Writings and Speeches of Martin Luther King Jr.*, ed. James Melvin Washington (New York: HarperSanFrancisco, 1991), 289.

9   Martin Luther King Jr., "Letter from Birmingham City Jail," in *Testament of Hope*, 289. It should be noted that King's direct–action tactics were unpopular with more than white clergy. According to Andrew Young, one of King's chief lieutenants, Thurgood Marshall preferred lawsuits

and legal strategies to change racially segregationist societal structures. Marshall was chief attorney for the Legal Defense Fund which
had successfully argued *Brown v. Topeka [Kansas] Board of Education*
ending separate but equal public schools. Young also noted that
during the Birmingham campaign, daily direct-action protests were
timed to end so film footage could be flown to New York in time to be
aired on nightly network news broadcasts. See Andrew Young, *An Easy
Burden: The Civil Rights Movement and the Transformation of America*
(New York: HarperCollins, 1996); Terri Laws, "Black Religion and Ideology in the Media: Birmingham 1963 Represented in Newsprint and
Television" (unpublished paper, May 10, 2009).

10   Martin Luther King Jr., interview on *Meet the Press*, April 17, 1960.

11   Philip Butler, *Black Transhuman Liberation Theology* (London: Bloomsbury, 2020), 38.

12   Butler, *Black Transhuman*, 32.

13   Butler, *Black Transhuman*, 38.

14   Luke 10:25–37.

15   The phrase is attributed to Cornel West.

16   Bart D. Ehrman, *The New Testament: A Historical Introduction to the
Early Christian Writings*, 3rd ed. (New York: Oxford University Press,
2004), 103–4.

17   Deirdre Cooper Owens, *Medical Bondage: Race, Gender, and the Origins
of American Gynecology* (Athens: University of Georgia Press, 2017),
16–19.

18   Esther Jones, "Africana Women's Science Fiction and Narrative Med-
icine: Difference, Ethics, and Empathy," in *Afrofuturism 2.0: The Rise of
Astro-Blackness*, ed. Reynaldo Anderson and Charles E. Jones (Lanham,
Md.: Lexington Books, 2016), 185.

19   Jones, "Africana," in Anderson and Jones, *Afrofuturism 2.0*, 186.

20   In the interest of space, I simply make note of Cuvier, who is lesser
known than Sims, but not so of his exploit. Cuvier is the scientist
behind the display of Sarah Baartman as a living, traveling exhibition.
Spectators lined up to examine her naked, exposed buttocks. When
she died, at only twenty-six years old, Cuvier dissected her body, giving particular attention to her labia and buttocks.

21   Vanessa Northington Gamble, "Under the Shadow of Tuskegee: African Americans and Health Care," *American Journal of Public Health* 87
(1997): 1773–78. See also L. L. Wall, "The Medical Ethics of Dr J Marion
Sims: A Fresh Look at the Historical Record," *Journal of Medical Ethics* 32
(2006): 346–50; and James Marion Sims, *Story of My Life*, ed. H. Marion
Sims (New York: D. Appleton, 1885), 241.

22   Sims, *Story*, 241. "The patient is not cured so long as there is the invol-
      untary loss of a single drop of urine. It would be tiresome for me to
      repeat in detail all the stages of improvement in the operation that
      were necessary before it was made perfect. These I have detailed in a
      surgical history of the facts, and to professional readers are still well
      known. Besides these three cases, I got three or four more to experi-
      ment on, and there was never a time that I could not, at any day, have
      had a subject for operation." Sims notes that he continued his exper-
      iments for four years.

23   Dennis Pillion, "Monument to 'Mothers of Gynecology' Unveiled in
      Montgomery," *AL.com*, September 27, 2021.

24   P. R. Lockhart, "New York Just Removed a Statue of a Surgeon Who
      Experimented on Enslaved Women," *Vox*, April 18, 2021, https://www
      .vox.com/identities/2018/4/18/17254234/j-marion-sims-experiments
      -slaves-women-gynecology-statue-removal. Sims' statue was relo-
      cated to the cemetery where he is buried.

25   Jane Akre, "AUGS Breaks with the Father of Gynecology," *Post and
      Courier*, July 4, 2018, https://www.meshmedicaldevicenewsdesk.com/
      articles/augs-breaks-with-the-father-of-gynecology.

26   Owens, *Medical Bondage*, 24

27   L. Lewis Wall, "The Medical Ethics of Dr J Marion Sims," *Journal of Med-
      ical Ethics* 32 (2006): 346–50.

28   Wall, "Medical Ethics," 346.

29   Wall, "Medical Ethics," 346.

30   Sims, *Story*, 241. The reader grasps her to be a white woman in that he
      uses the prefix "Mrs." with her last name, and attributes sympathies to
      the hardscrabble life she leads.

31   Sims, *Story*, 228.

32   Owens, *Medical Bondage*, 19. Owens observes that the term began to
      be used to describe poor immigrant white women in the late nine-
      teenth century, well after the end of legal U.S. slavery; the economic
      incentive tied to enslavement in the birthing of another future laborer
      was also clearly different. See p. 20.

33   Randall McLaughlin, "The Birth of a Nation: A Study of Slavery in
      Seventeenth-Century Virginia," *Hastings Race and Poverty Law Jour-
      nal* 16, no. 1 (2019), https://repository.uchastings.edu/hastings_race
      _poverty_law_journal/vol16/iss1/2.

34   Owens, *Medical Bondage*, 11.

35   Sims, *Story*, 251.

36 Famous cases include the minimization of Serena Williams' postdelivery story. She previously had an embolism. Knowing this, when she began to feel unwell, she requested blood thinners. Refusal to hear her concerns resulted in multiple postdelivery surgeries to rid her body of numerous, life-threatening blood clots. Serena Williams, "How Serena Williams Saved Her Own Life," *Elle*, April 5, 2022, https://www.elle.com/life-love/a39586444/how-serena-williams-saved-her-own-life/.

37 Kelli M. Hoffman, Sophie Trawalter, Jordan R. Axt, and M. Norman Oliver, "Racial Bias in Pain Assessment and Treatment Recommendations, and False Beliefs about Biological Differences between Blacks and Whites," *Proceedings of the National Academy of the Sciences of the United States of America* 113, no. 16 (2016): 4296–301, www.pnas.org/cgi/doi/10.1073/pnas.1516047113.

38 Jones, "Africana," in Anderson and Jones, *Afrofuturism 2.0*, 189.

39 Jones, "Africana," in Anderson and Jones, *Afrofuturism 2.0*, 195.

40 Butler, *Black Transhuman*, 40.

41 Butler, *Black Transhuman*, 40.

42 Butler, *Black Transhuman*, 40.

43 Cone's contributions to theological method appear in his groundbreaking works within the discipline. This has led many scholars to refer to him as the "father of Black Theology." Those works are James H. Cone, *Black Theology and Black Power* (Maryknoll, N.Y.: Orbis Books, 1969) and James H. Cone, *A Black Theology of Liberation* (Maryknoll, N.Y.: Orbis Books, 1970). See the chapter conclusion for additional comments.

44 Space does not allow for a full treatment of human flourishing of my interest here. See Miroslav Volf, Matthew Croasmun, and Ryan McAnnally-Linz, "Meanings and Dimensions of Flourishing: A Programmatic Sketch," in *Religion and Human Flourishing*, ed. Adam B. Cohen (Waco, Tex.: Baylor University Press, 2020), 7–17.

45 Rob Stein, "A Young Mississippi Woman's Journey through a Pioneering Gene-Editing Experiment," *All Things Considered*, National Public Radio, December 25, 2019, https://www.npr.org/sections/health-shots/2019/12/25/784395525/a-young-mississippi-womans-journey-through-a-pioneering-gene-editing-experiment.

46 "What Is Sickle Cell Disease?" National Heart, Lung, and Blood Institute, https://www.nhlbi.nih.gov/health/sickle-cell-disease.

47 When adult sickle cell patients are in crisis, they often must go to an emergency room in search of pain relief. The medical establishment is notorious for presuming that these encounters are a ruse for patients seeking drugs rather than pain treatment. For a book-length treatment of the life of sickle cell patients, especially making the transition

from pediatric to adult medicine, see Carolyn Moxley Rouse, *Uncertain Suffering: Racial Health Care Disparities and Sickle Cell Disease* (Berkeley: University of California Press, 2009).

48   Rob Stein, "In a 1st, Doctors in U.S. Use CRISPR Tool to Treat Patient with Genetic Disorder," *Morning Edition*, National Public Radio, July 29, 2019, https://www.npr.org/sections/health-shots/2019/07/29/744826505/ sickle-cell-patient-reveals-why-she-is-volunteering-for-landmark -gene-editing-st.

49   This is not to suggest that Black bodies are biologically different than other bodies. Rather, this comment regarding the lack of sustained attention to Black inequity is factual relative to a host of issues in Black life, including socioeconomic and political concerns as well as health inequity.

50   For a salient example to understand its legacy, see F. N. Boney, ed., *A Slave Life in Georgia: A Narrative of the Life, Sufferings, and Escape of John Brown, a Fugitive Slave* (Savannah, Ga.: Beehive Press, 1972).

9

DISABILITY JUSTICE, BIOENHANCEMENT, AND THE ESCHATOLOGICAL IMAGINATION

Devan Stahl

Eschatology is a powerful site for thinking about disability because it calls us to consider what place we hold for disability in our imagined futures whether that future cradles or erases disability, how we imagine liberation might one day unfold for us, the taste of it, how it feels against the skin.[1]

Christians and transhumanists alike long for a world in which bodies and societies are radically transformed. These eschatological imaginings often portray disabled bodies as unfit for the future. Understanding disability as something inherently bad, many Christians and transhumanists seek to fix or eradicate disability to signal or even usher in the future they hope for. The erasure of disabled bodies from religious and secular eschatologies, however, results from and can lead to eugenic practices that violate the integrity of disabled bodies, fail to acknowledge the value and moral worth of disabled people, and reinscribe ableist structures and practices. Insofar as Christians and transhumanists believe they can participate in the future societies they long for, each must carefully consider the relationship between justice and disability.

This chapter places bioethicists, disability and crip scholars, and Christian ethicists into conversation concerning how to frame justice within bioenhancement debates. Bioethicists, who remain split

206 | Devan Stahl

on whether enhancement technologies ought to be pursued, commonly question how bioenhancement technologies can be developed and distributed ethically as well as how to ensure persons with disabilities are not further disadvantaged when enhancements become prevalent. Justice within these debates is often framed as enhancing equality of opportunity through bioenhancements so that those who are disadvantaged because of the genetic lottery can fully participate in society. Disability advocates, on the other hand, argue that institutional structures and not individual bodies should be the target of enhancement. Justice requires recognition of the value of disabled people[2] and their contributions to society. Crip scholars build off and at times challenge this thinking, imagining a future in which the idea of the "normal body" is undermined and disability is seen as potentially desirable. Within this crip future, bioenhancement technologies have a place, insofar as they enable people to fit their bodies to their environments while also celebrating their bodily diversity.

To assess the ethics of bioenhancement technologies, Christian ethicists should take note of the justice arguments made by transhumanists, bioethicists, and disability scholars. Rather than insulate itself from secular discourse, Christians ought to carefully consider the critiques leveled by disability scholars that ableism shapes the ways modern people imagine equality within the present and the future. It might be that ableism has obstructed modern Christians from properly interpreting the scriptural promises of eternal life with God. Purged of its own ableism, Christian ethicists can then add to conversations and critiques of our transhuman future a compelling account of kingdom-oriented justice that includes disabled people within the body of Christ. Mutual dialogue between bioethicists, disability and crip scholars, and Christian ethicists can enhance conversations concerning the place of disability in our imagined futures.

JUSTICE WITHIN THE BIOETHICS DEBATES

As has become clear in previous chapters, ontological and teleological questions are inherent within bioenhancement debates. The transhumanist goal of becoming "posthuman" or "human plus" implies there is something wrong or lacking in our current embodiment. For transhumanists, the limited and finite nature of our bodies prevents us from pursuing certain goals that would require a longer life span, greater cognitive capacity, and even superior moral capacities. Physical, cognitive, and moral enhancements seek to overcome the natural limitations of individual bodies with the goal of fostering individual as well as communal well-being.

Given the overarching goals of transhumanists, questions of justice are integral to bioenhancement debates. Depending on how we evaluate the ontology and teleology of enhancement projects, enhancements might be understood as important for the common good. People who are physically enhanced may be in a better position to contribute to the flourishing of industry, the economy, or protection of the state through military service. People who are cognitively enhanced may be in a better position to develop scientific breakthroughs, novel technologies, or political strategies that help to solve dilemmas facing our global community. Those who are morally enhanced might make better moral choices, help other humans, and care for the natural environment.

The potential for enhancement technologies to affect the flourishing of humans and the natural world leads thinkers to consider how *developing* them falls within the realm of justice. The development of bioenhancement technologies will require considerable resources, including financial resources from private companies and possibly the federal government,[3] as well as investments of time and energy by researchers. The costs of developing bioenhancements are likely to be substantial and, therefore, must be justified by the potential they have to improve the lives of individuals as well as society.

One of the major justice concerns raised by critics is that enhancements will do little to address health disparities across the population. Many fear that vast healthcare disparities are likely to be replicated or even exacerbated through bioenhancement technologies. It is no wonder, then, that persons coming from underrepresented minority groups—such as women, racial and ethnic minorities, and people with disabilities—are skeptical that bioenhancement technologies will be developed and distributed fairly. If we wish to create societies in which all human beings can flourish, technologies aimed at enhancing individuals must also consider the common good and work toward equity. For example, invest-ments in radical life extension do nothing to address the health disparities that result in shorter life expectancies for historically marginalized groups.[4] Focusing on individual biology neglects the social determinants of health, which have a far greater impact on overall health and lifespan, not to mention people's ability to pur-sue life goals.

To respond to this critique, some bioethicists and most trans-humanists have argued that physical enhancements ought to be coupled with cognitive and moral enhancements to ensure tech-nologies will be developed fairly.[5] We can achieve equity by invest-ing in biotechnologies that improve the cognitive capacities of people trying to find innovative solutions to health disparities, or, as some have proposed, technologies themselves might eliminate cognitive biases or problematic emotional states (e.g., race aversion) that justify such disparities.[6] If we imagine that bioenhancement technologies could produce these promised outcomes for individ-uals and for society (and there is reason to be skeptical of many such claims),[7] then the question becomes one of just *distribution* of enhancements.

At present, most biomedical interventions that are considered "enhancements" (e.g., cosmetic plastic surgery to improve appear-ance or synthetic hormones to improve athletic performance or physique) are not typically covered by insurance in the United States or by national health insurance programs in the United Kingdom and elsewhere.[8] At least initially, it is likely that bioenhancement tech-nologies will be prohibitively expensive for most people. Thus, many bioethicists worry that bioenhancements will only exacerbate social inequalities.[9] Moral and cognitive enhancements might prompt their users to work toward remedying current inequalities, but this would be only a potential downstream side effect. If enhancements achieve their intended purpose, those who can afford to be physi-cally or cognitively enhanced will have distinct advantages over the unenhanced, and those who experience inequities would be at the benevolent mercy of the already enhanced.

Humanity+ (also known as the World Transhumanist Associa-tion) admits that initially bioenhancement technologies will benefit the rich and widen social inequalities. Those who are already wealthy will be able to afford technologies that increase their physical and cognitive capacities and those of their children, likely leading to further wealth accumulation for those at the top of the socioeconomic ladder.[10] Humanity+ claims this probable reality is no reason to ban bioenhancement technologies, however, because history shows that medicines and consumer electronics eventually become more affordable as they become more routine. "Even in the poorest countries, millions of people have benefited from vaccines and penicillin. . . . The price of computers and other devices that were once cutting-edge only a couple of years ago drops precipitously as new models are introduced."[11] Income distribution is a "political problem," but technological progress eventually helps all people by increasing resources to all.[12] In other words, the rising tide of technology lifts all boats.

Bioethicists have critiqued this trickle-down, market-based approach to the fair distribution of bioenhancement technologies arguing that bioenhancements ought to be distributed in such a way that they target those who are most disadvantaged in society. Egalitarians who promote the fair equality of opportunity, for example, argue that if they are not distributed fairly, enhancements will further compromise the equality of opportunities available to people.[13] It is not fair, they claim, that some people are disadvantaged through the so-called natural lottery—some people are simply not as smart or physically able as others. Although no person or institution is responsible for producing inborn disadvantages, most egalitarians believe it is still the responsibility of the state to create a level playing field for all.

Of course, there are multiple ways the state might level the playing field. If one believes, however, that abilities and other inborn qualities create unfair advantages and disadvantages in life, it might make sense to offer to subsidize enhancements to some, while barring others from receiving enhancements. Bioethicists Alberto Giubilini and Francesca Minerva suggest that those who are the most disadvantaged in society (e.g., the disabled and the poor) should receive subsidies to pay for enhancements and those who are born into the most favorable social and economic conditions should be prohibited from receiving enhancements.[14] They argue that enhancements can produce equality of opportunity by ensuring that only those who are most negatively affected by their genetic, biological, and social circumstances are enhanced.[15] Not all bioethicists agree with this heavy-handed approach to fair distribution, but many do believe that bioenhancement technologies, if distributed fairly, can reduce inequalities through biological improvements.

DISABILITY JUSTICE

Of course, it is exactly this targeting of biology to solve social inequalities that rankles many disability scholars and activists. Egalitarians rarely claim that other minority communities must undergo biological changes to achieve justice. Many bioethicists, particularly those who promote enhancement technologies, seem to take it for granted that disability is an inherently negative or even harmful biological characteristic. (This has become known as the "standard view" among disability bioethicists.)[16] For decades, disability advocates have been arguing that disability results from the interaction between a person and his or her social and physical environment. Many of the disadvantages that people with disabilities experience stem from social barriers and standards of normalcy rather than biological impairments. Fair distribution of resources, therefore, cannot simply target individual bodies but must also include the modification of social structures.

Many Christians also understand disability as an ontological deficiency rather than primarily as a problem of social barriers and attitudes. Many theologians presume prelapsarian bodies were perfect and incorruptible and, therefore, any marker of finitude or limitation is a direct result of human sinfulness.[17] Disabilities are therefore understood as intimately connected to original sin—it is only through the fall that bodies can become disabled. Disability theologians often reject this connection, however, arguing that limitation and finitude are a natural part of the human condition and not the result of original sin.[18] As long as sin and disability are easily correlated, those who are considered victims of the natural lottery either will provoke moral revulsion or will become the focus of intensive efforts aimed at spiritual or medical cure. Rather than locating sin in individual bodies, disability theologians believe sin occurs when nondisabled persons alienate and ostracize people with disabilities. Sin is the result of our failure to be in proper relationship with ourselves, one another, and God. By taking up a *social model* of disability, many disability theologians see sin as tied to structures and attitudes that isolate and exclude people with disabilities.

Most enhancement proponents, on the other hand, promote a *medical model* of disability, arguing that disabilities are a "lack of certain basic sensory, physical, or cognitive capacities" that reduce "a broad range of valuable options and opportunities."[19] To have a fair share of opportunity "requires a minimum level of cognitive capacities, physical abilities, and some desirable social traits, such as empathy and agreeableness."[20] It is not clear, however, that biological impairments—as opposed to architecture, attitudes, and standards of normalcy—are the reason that people with disabilities lack opportunities in society. A lower-than-average IQ may lead to "domination, exclusion, lower income, deprivation, and low self-esteem,"[21] as Giubilini and Minerva claim, but it does not follow that one's problem is one's IQ score and not a system that valorizes certain cognitive capacities above all else. Moreover, it is far from clear that lacking a higher-than-average IQ results in failure to achieve a "decent minimum quality of life,"[22] as Giubilini and Minerva claim, unless a high quality of life requires entrance into a top university as they suggest. (In fact, there is good reason to believe that general happiness is not closely associated with attendance at elite universities.)[23]

Enhancement proponents tie well-being so closely to an abundance of life options that it becomes impossible to believe that any human could thrive without an infinitely wide range of opportunities.[24] Disability advocates also recognize that discriminatory attitudes and a lack of accommodations in employment, education, and other sectors unfairly limit life options for people with disabilities. Yet "choice," or the availability of an infinite number of opportunities in life, is not the only or even primary driver of well-being. There are many things that might enable us to have a good life. Choice, in and of itself, is not necessarily good; rather, choice is good when it allows us access to opportunities that will enable us to thrive.

Against those who claim that disabilities inherently diminish one's opportunities in life as well as well-being, many disability scholars argue disabilities ought to be understood as intrinsically neutral.[25] Disabilities, in and of themselves, are not necessarily bad for a person apart from the context in which people find themselves. This is not to say that most people experience disability as neutral. Disability almost certainly affects well-being, but disabilities do not predetermine one's well-being, nor are they singularly or overwhelmingly responsible for well-being. The goodness or badness of any particular disability for any particular person rests upon how an individual responds to her disability, how she interacts with her environment, the social attitudes and barriers she may experience, and pure accident of circumstance.[26] It would, therefore, be inappropriate to claim that disability always makes a person worse off or that the best or only way to increase well-being is to eliminate disability. Justice does not require that we eliminate disabilities; rather, it requires that we identify and correct the circumstances that truly disadvantage disabled people.

Many disability scholars look beyond *distributive justice* to secure social equality for people with disabilities. Whereas bioenhancement proponents focus on how to fairly distribute resources, disability advocates are equally interested in *recognitive justice*, which seeks to secure equal respect for all individuals.[27] Respecting individuals demands that we understand and work toward their self-identified interests. Rarely do enhancement proponents cite disability scholars or surveys of people with disabilities to understand their desire for enhancement technologies, much less how they should be developed or distributed. In fact, bioethicists consistently reject evidence that people with physical and cognitive disabilities already rate their quality of life as equal to that of nondisabled people.[28]

The lack of attention to, or outright dismissal of, the justice concerns of disability scholars and activists results in a narrow conception of the good that demands certain biological capacities to achieve well-being. As a result, bioenhancement proponents seek first to eradicate rather than accommodate disability. This is perhaps clearest when proponents endorse eugenic solutions to the problem of disability in utero.

Many proponents of human enhancement readily admit that eugenic selection is the best way to achieve human enhancement.[29] Parents already have the option of selecting against genetic disability through selective abortion and preimplantation genetic screenings, which many disability advocates believe can further stigmatize disability by reducing well-being to genotype. Not only do bioenhancement proponents see disability as opposed to well-being, but they also tend to see genetic markers and predispositions as a stand-in for disability. Some enhancement proponents have even gone so far as to argue that "morally conscientious" parents should not allow children with genetic markers for disability to be born and that once enhancements are safe, they ought to become compulsory, "like education or fluoride in the water."[30]

Genetic engineering might one day allow parents to not only select against genetic markers for disability but also select for (or even build in) enhanced traits. Enhanced children will not only lack disabilities, but they would also have "superior" traits. One prominent transhumanist has even gone so far as to argue that "germ-line enhancement will lead to more love and parental dedication. Some mothers and fathers might find it easier to love a child who, thanks to enhancements, is bright, beautiful, healthy, and happy."[31] Of course, there is little evidence that parents of disabled children love or appreciate them less.[32] Such overt disability discrimination and acceptance of eugenics is unlikely to find support among disability advocates.

Unfortunately, Christian churches have not been pillars of accommodation for people with disabilities, nor do they always provide places for them to flourish. In fact, many predominantly white mainline denominations were enthusiastic supporters of eugenic programs in the early twentieth century, and few have apologized for their eager promotion of eugenic sterilization.[33] Religious leaders also fought to be exempt from ADA requirements of accessibility, and many still struggle with creating spaces and worship styles that fully include people with disabilities into the life of their congregations. Yet, if Christians wish to embody their relationship with God through their worship or liturgy, they must create spaces where they, in the words of disability theologian Rebecca Spurrier, "rehearse a Christian response to an encounter with the creative beauty of divine love, which makes possible belonging to a community through and across difference."[34] Inclusive practices honor the creative beauty of God and God's creation. This embrace of difference and creativity is taken up with crip scholarship.

CRIP JUSTICE

The proposition that justice ought to be achieved through the eradication of future disabled persons will not find much support among disability advocates, but this does not mean that people with disabilities will outright reject all enhancement technologies. Crip scholars have extended the conversation of justice to include recognition of the generative aspects of disability, including the creation of biotechnologies. Crip (short for "cripple"—a reclaiming of what has become derogatory slang) scholarship seeks to disrupt the fixed categories of "disabled" and "nondisabled" and instead discuss "collective affinities" of people with various body-minds, impairments, and illnesses, who are disabled or nonnormal.[35] Crip scholars imagine a more expansive disability movement that allows those without impairments to also identify as disabled (e.g., the Hearing Children of Deaf Adults and the lovers and friends of those who are disabled) and acknowledges the multiple and inter-sectional identities of people with disabilities (e.g., gender, sex-ual orientation, race, ethnicity, etc.).[36] Given this more expansive understanding of who counts as disabled, posthumans and other enhanced persons may also be understood as disabled—persons with unusual body-minds who have nonstandard and yet desir-able bodies. Of course, most transhumanists are likely to reject referring to the posthuman body as disabled, but that is because they adhere to a medical model of disability that understands dis-ability as an *inherent lack* rather than a crip understanding of *non-normative embodiment*. Crip scholars challenge transhumanists to expand their notions of normativity and disability.

Crip scholars imagine a just future as one in which nonconfor-mity and diversity are celebrated rather than merely accommodated or compensated for, through the fair distribution of resources. For many crip scholars, the common good is advanced by recognizing not only the humanity and moral worth of people with disabilities but the generative creativity that stems from persons with nonnormative body-minds. Persons with physical, sensory, and neurocognitive dis-abilities continually invent unusual ways to function in society.

Crip scholars share with transhumanists an openness toward cutting-edge biotechnologies and an expansive imagination for what constitutes the human form. From wheelchairs to prosthetics to neural implants, many people with disabilities have adopted technologies that alter their bodies to fit their environment. With transhumanists, many disabled people can easily imagine an embodied life wherein the demarcations between organism and machine blur. As Donna Haraway articulates in "A Cyborg Manifesto," in late modernity we are all hybrids.[37] The neat divisions we have created between the "natural" and the "artificial" have always been tenuous. This has only become truer in the decades since Haraway's manifesto. Our smart phones, for example, which seem to be always at our fingertips, extend our cognitive and communicative capacities. In fact, many of the current technologies we enjoy were first created for or by people with disabilities seeking to increase their physical, sensory, or cognitive functionality (e.g., screen readers, speech recognition software, eye-gaze tracking, cleaning robots, talking elevators, curb cuts, etc.). Disability has been generative of many technologies that are useful to disabled and nondisabled people alike. This is sometimes referred to as the *Curb-Cut Effect*.

Bioenhancement proponents are right to point out that, perhaps more than any other group, people with disabilities are open to integrating technology into their bodies. The enhancement of bodies need not merely increase functionality, however. In the dance performance *Where Good Souls Fear*, for example, disabled dancer Alice Sheppard is seen in a wheelchair using forearm crutches. She writes:

> In the world of impairment functional design no one needs both kinds of mobility technologies at once. In fact, this doubling of technology rather denies its functional purpose in that it significantly restricts movement. In this form, mine is a disabled body disarticulated from medical need. . . . This body is supplicant only to desire and a simultaneous urge to revel in the excess of disability.[38]

For many disability scholars and advocates, assistive technologies celebrate bodily diversity, understanding the disabled body as generative rather than deviant. The acceptance and celebration of difference within crip scholarship and activism can occur with or without technology.

Although crip scholars and transhumanists share the language of the "posthuman" body, their understanding of this body is radically divergent, in part because they imagine the future differently. Even though many people with disabilities (although certainly not all) readily embrace assistive technologies, they do not all share transhumanists' seeming disgust with the limitation and vulnerability of human bodies or the hierarchies of ability that devalue people with intellectual disabilities. Most transhumanists clearly create a mind–body dualism that favors the mind. Nick Bostrom, for example, refers to the human body as a "self–combusting paper hut" that must be overcome if humans wish to feel secure in life.[39] Ray Kurzweil imagines that one day humans will adopt virtual, indestructible forms of life by uploading their consciousness into computers and living in simulated, virtual bodies.[40] Persons using assistive technologies do not necessarily share the desire to be rid of their physical bodies altogether. Moreover, many people who use assistive technologies do not understand those technologies as helping to overcome disability. Wheelchairs, for example, do not render their users nondisabled, although they do enhance mobility.

Even at its most radical, the imagined posthuman body described by transhumanists seems to reify rather than undermine the hyper–able and hyper–masculine body that transhumanists admire. In his paper, "Why I Want to Be a Posthuman When I Grow Up," Nick Bostrom describes the posthuman body as active, productive, intellectually capable of understanding and appreciating music and mathematics, stronger, more energetic, younger, funnier, more able to appreciate Proust, more likely to play jazz than watch television, more likely to play virtual reality games with friends than watch sports, and more likely to support charity work for animals than hang out at a pub. Bostrom highlights not only the capacities he values (e.g., cognitive ability) but even his unique aesthetic tastes and activities.

Clearly, our future imaginaries reveal our desires and our values. Bostrom's posthuman, with his appetite for the "high arts" and penchant for giving to charitable causes, resembles a kind of upper–middle–class white savior. His vision of the enhanced human is a far cry from Donna Haraway's hybrid cyborg, Sheppard's (dis) functional crutch wearer, or the wounded body of Christ. Christian theologians ought to respond to the idealized body and communities being imagined by both transhumanists and crip scholars. With transhumanists, Christians might want to emphasize the resurrected body in the kingdom of God as overcoming certain aspects of our current embodied lives. The kingdom is a place wherein God will dwell with humans, and their pain and suffering will be no more:

> See, the home of God is among mortals.
> He will dwell with them;
> They will be his peoples,
> And God himself will be with them;
> He will wipe every tear from their eyes.
> Death will be no more;
> Mourning and crying and pain will be no more,
> For the first things have passed away. (Rev 21:3–4, NRSV)

At the same time, Christian eschatology does not promise the kind of immortality promised by transhumanists; in the kingdom of God, finite human life does not cease to be finite; rather, it is "taken into" the infinite, eternal life of God. In other words, God clothes our mortality with immortality (1 Cor 15:53). With crip scholars, Christians might imagine the kingdom not as a place where all bodies become super-able or hypernormalized but as a place in which people are invited to feast together just as they are (Luke 14:13–23). Just as the bread of the Eucharist does not cease to be bread when it becomes the body of Christ but becomes more fully itself, so too might persons with disabilities become more of what they are without ceasing to be themselves. In the kingdom, bodies are simultaneously transformed and identifiable (1 Cor 15:36–45). Unlike either transhumanists or crip scholars, however, Christians believe the norm for this body will be Christ's own resurrected body. Bodies will be christo-formed (1 Cor 15:45–57; 1 John 3:2). Christ's body was simultaneously glorified and wounded, bearing the marks of his crucifixion. The Christian "posthuman" body will resemble Christ's own resurrected body and the kingdom he imagined wherein the "poor, the crippled, the blind, and the lame" are invited to feast at tables of honor (Luke 14:21).

In juxtaposing crip and Christian imaginaries with the posthuman body of transhumanism, we move beyond a focus on justice as equality to the idea of justice as superabundance. By restricting justice conversations to the distribution of resources, the creative and pleasurable aspects of our future life are left by the wayside. The crip imaginary presses Christians to imagine a future in which our concept of justice is itself enhanced and our ideal future is not simply a space in which each is given their just deserts. With disability and crip scholars, we may begin to consider the kingdom of God as more dynamic and radically transformed than we had previously imagined. The kingdom of God is not merely a place wherein each is given what they are due but a place in which well-being includes creative, pleasurable, and interdependent forms of life.

Transhumanism and Christian Eschatology

Crip scholars' emphasis on the future of nonnormative embodiment should stretch Christians to consider disability within their own eschatological imaginings. All too often, Christians imagine the kingdom as a perfected version of their particular and historically situated society rather than as a radical transformation of the current world order. Despite biblical warnings that we cannot know how our bodies will appear in the resurrection (1 John 3:1–3), Christians are prone to understand bodies within this kingdom as normalized rather than transformed. Christian theologians have long imagined the kingdom of God as a place where defects and disabilities are eliminated. Although the exact visions of the resurrected body differ, what most theologians have agreed upon is that resurrected bodies in the kingdom will be free of blemishes, defects, and disabilities.[41] The very characteristics that people with disabilities value about their embodiment are targeted as bodily states that will be "fixed" in the resurrection. If the kingdom of God is a place that eradicates disability, however, it may also eradicate individual experience and pride. Recognizing that resurrected bodies bear some resemblance to Christ's resurrected body, some disability theologians have countered the idea that resurrected bodies are "blemish-free" by noting Christ's own resurrected body displayed the marks of his crucifixion (John 20:27).[42]

Rather than an idealized or normalized body, disability theologians encourage us to imagine a kingdom in which disabilities remain but their associated impairments are mitigated. Nancy

Eiesland, Amos Yong, and Richard Cross rebut the idea that disabled bodies will be cured or fixed in the kingdom. Nancy Eiesland, for example, recalls being told as a child that in heaven she would no longer limp. Rather than a hopeful promise, however, Eiesland worried God would not know who she was if her limp was taken away. Eiesland counters the typical Christian understanding of disability in the kingdom by arguing that her disabilities are part of her identity, and if they were not present in heaven, then she could not know herself and likewise could not be known by God.[43] Amos Yong likewise speculates that people with disabilities will not be awarded the powerful and beautiful bodies that Western culture prizes; rather, they will retain their self-identity and perhaps even their phenotypical features. Persons with disabilities will experience individual and corporate transformation such that they will be recognized for their proper role in God's natural order and within the communion of saints.[44] Using the work of Duns Scotus, Richard Cross suggests disabilities are purposefully created by God, who finds beauty in disability. In the resurrection, bodily impairments would be accommodated such that persons can achieve their teleological ends (suggesting that the environment and not the impairment is the problem).[45] As with contemporary crip scholars, Scotus' connection between the aesthetic aspects of life and his ethics provides him a more expansive understanding of the goods of disability than other theologians.[46]

It is not wrong in principle that we seek to mitigate or even eliminate certain effects of human limitation, particularly limitations that separate us from God and cause us harm. And of course, medicine and technoscience can play a role in creating the godly and just society we imagine within the kingdom of God. Along with disability and crip scholars, Christians should neither fully embrace the medical model of disability nor reject all medical interventions upon disabled bodies. If the kingdom is a place in which pain and suffering will be no more, eradicating pain and suffering can give us a glimpse of our future state. But we should not assume all disabilities cause pain and suffering. Our eschatological imaginations can accommodate technoscience, as long as the technology developed does not attempt to eradicate or overcome the disabled body. Technologies made for people with disabilities signal (though will certainly not supplant or stand in for) our ultimate hopes for disabled bodies: either through elimination or celebration. Disability-friendly, eschatologically informed technologies can exist, but only within certain parameters.

What would constitute a "disability-friendly, eschatologically informed" bioenhancement? Two kinds of technologies meant for persons with disabilities can evoke notions of the future, posthuman body: the exoskeleton and the endoskeletal prosthesis. Both exoskeletons and prostheses purport to enhance functionality and improve quality of life, yet they have notable differences. The goal of the exoskeleton is to eradicate disability, enabling its wearer to have "normal" interactions. Standing and walking are seen as obviously superior to sitting and wheeling, and so quality of life is expected to improve using an exoskeleton. The prosthesis, however, allows its user to carry out his or her goals, which are varied, through the use of assistive technology, which often can be swapped out as the user desires, making the wearer what Sharon Betcher calls a "prosthetic erratic."[47] Whereas the exoskeleton attempts to normalize the body (which is ironic since the exoskeleton is immediately obvious and inorganic), a certain type of prosthesis can enhance disability through its functional and aesthetic qualities.

The Exoskeleton as a Site of Violence and Domination

Robotic exoskeletons are "wearable robotic units controlled by computer boards to power a system of motors, pneumatics, levers, or hydraulics to restore [or enhance] locomotion."[48] They are now advertised as solutions to the "problem" of paralysis, but paraplegics were an afterthought to the design of these exoskeletons. The U.S. military first began to develop exoskeletons in the 1960s, partnering with General Electric on Hardiman (Human Augmentation Research and Development Investigation).[49] The idea was to give soldiers a boost when running and carrying heavy equipment. In the early 2000s, exoskeletons were developed for factory workers who needed to carry large loads over long distances.[50] Many technologies used to enable persons with disabilities to gain access to our society were initially designed through military-industrial research.

Once tech companies set their sights on paraplegics, they reinforced the cultural narrative about the pitiable cripple to sell their products. As Brian Brock previously described, biotech companies positioned themselves as benevolent saviors, enabling wearers to overcome the confines of the traditional wheelchair. In a tweet from Ekso Bionics advertising their newest exoskeleton, you see an empty wheelchair in a rehab clinic. Barely visible on the right side of the image is a person standing. The tagline reads, "Sometimes, care lives in an empty wheelchair."[51] The care taken by the rehabilitation specialist, not to mention the device user, is glossed over in favor of the exoskeleton itself as care-provider.

Another ad for an exoskeleton created by Ekso Bionics depicts a young, normative-looking white man pictured in five panes, moving from his wheelchair into a standing and walking position.[52] The image is clearly an analogy to the "march of progress" images that illustrate the evolution of *Homo sapiens* over twenty-five million years. The message is obvious: standing is progress from sitting. Man (nearly all the ads will feature white men) is meant to stand. The upright man is thus the apex of progress, and the exoskeleton is "not merely revolutionary, but evolutionary, not only desirable but inevitable."[53]

Within discussions of the exoskeleton, the triumphalist narrative concerning disability remains untouched: the pitiable paralyzed man can now pull himself up by his robotic bootstraps to walk like a "normal" person. The tech industry describes exoskeletons as "helping the infirm" form "greater independence and quality of life" and "break out of the 'wheel-chair bubble.'"[54] Other companies describe the machines as "miracles" akin to healing narratives in the Bible.[55] Ironically, this picturesque image of disability eliminated obscures the underlying ontology of the body in the exoskeleton, which is violence and efficiency. While most tech companies are developing exoskeletons for both military and rehab purposes, the focus of their public advertising is on their biomedical use.

The exoskeleton was clearly developed using a medical model of disability that demands that bodies, and not external environments, must change for persons with disabilities to be accommodated. The imperative to fix disability requires an overcoming of paralysis to fit into ableist ideals of "normal" mobility. American transhumanist Zolton Istvan argues societies should invest in exoskeletons rather than communal infrastructure. In arguing against a court order that required Los Angeles to invest $1.3 billion in sidewalks and access ways, Istvan declared we should leave sidewalks in disrepair and instead "repair physically disabled human beings, and make them mobile and able-bodied again."[56] Repairing sidewalks, which of course disabled and nondisabled people use, is part of American "bandage culture" that fails to eliminate the "root of the problem"[57] (i.e., disability). As a presidential candidate, Istvan vowed to eliminate disability through technology and modern medicine.

The Prosthesis as a Site for Christian Eschatological Justice

For many disability advocates, exoskeletons represent a harmful, violent, medicalized view of disability. All too often, engineers, working without input from persons with mobility impairments, make top-down assumptions about what people with disabilities desire. In opposition to this practice, designers, artists, and disabled people sometimes collaborate to create new forms of biotechnology. Such collaborations often aim at resisting the normalizing tendencies of assistive technologies. Innovations in endoskeletal prostheses are alternatives to the exoskeleton. As with exoskeletons, prostheses seek to enhance the functionality of persons with mobility impairments; unlike exoskeletons, however, prostheses can (when justly created) seek to celebrate rather than overcome disability.

The collaborative biotechnologies I describe below are a potent site for the realization of crip justice for the Christian eschatological imaginary. Drawing upon the insights of crip techno-scholars, I propose four criteria that disability theologians can use to assess whether biotechnologies can enrich crip eschatology. Just prosthetics ought to be (1) person-centered, (2) queer, (3) dynamic, and (4) relational.

First, eschatologically oriented biotech should be person-centered. The goal of biotechnologies should not be to "fix" or normalize the individual wearer but to create dynamic partnerships wherein people with disabilities are seen as having critical knowledge to contribute to biotechnologies. Including disabled people in creative projects may produce structural change as well as improved products for individuals. Of course, people with disabilities are themselves subject to the same lures of normalization that are prevalent in our society. Internalized ableism may distort even

the desires of disabled people. It is certainly possible for a prosthesis to aim at the erasure of disability for the sake of normalization of capitalist efficiency. Yet, without the input of disabled people, technologies designed for them will certainly fail to meet their
most basic needs. The result is often technologies that cause pain,
have undesirable side effects, are prohibitively expensive, or are built
merely to make the nondisabled more comfortable with the disabled people they encounter.

Crip technoscience, on the other hand, is committed to centering disabled people as agents of technoscience rather than mere
consumers. This is to suggest not that agency in and of itself is a
prevailing good but that including disabled people in the design
of their own prosthetics is a bare minimum for ethical creation.
By privileging people with disabilities as knowers and creators, we
can undermine the social systems that exclude and oppress them.
Eschatologically oriented technologies must resist the normalization of bodies as well as the notion that disabled people must first
be fixed to contribute to society.

Person-centered technologies were on full display in 2016,
when the White House hosted the Design for All showcase, which
exhibited inclusive fashionwear, assistive technologies, and prostheses designed and worn by disabled people. In the showcase,
disability was celebrated as a source of creativity and not a medical problem to be fixed or cured. In the showcase, Peregrine, who
works with the global e-NABLE community of prosthetic designers
and developers, proclaimed, "I wear this hand because I designed
it, I made it, and it's me."[58] Peregrine's prosthetic is not a product
meant to fix their body; it is an innovative and collaborative project
that celebrates their body, knowledge, and ingenuity. Through Peregrine's creation and exclamation, we may be prompted to imagine a kingdom in which disability is celebrated as a site for creative
relationality.

In addition to being functional, disability engineers and artists
also create assistive technologies that are *queer*, or nonnormative, creative, pleasurable, and communal. Lisa Bufano, a bilateral
amputee, for example, created prosthetic legs she says feel both
pleasing and comfortable.[59] In one of her most famous works,
Bufano wears prosthetic stilts she made from twenty-eight-inch

curved table legs. Working outside of biomedicine, Bufano's legs are created for pleasurable play rather than exclusively for her functionality or capitalist efficiency. Bufano also invites her collaborator, Sonsherée Giles, a non-amputee, to wear the stilts, raising questions about who prosthetics are for.[60] In the kingdom of God, our bodies may be transformed in ways in which the dichotomy between disabled and nondisabled are no longer relevant. Compulsory able-bodiedness does not exist in this kingdom; instead, disability is a creative and generative embodiment that allows for unusual relations.

Kingdom-inspired biotech should also be *dynamic*. Rather than static, normalized, or idealized bodies, we might imagine our resurrected bodies are continually transforming as we relate to God, one another, and ourselves. Dynamic biotechnologies honor the ever-changing nature of bodies, which result from natural biological processes as well as the changing nature of what constitutes the "normal" body.[61] Not all bodily changes in this life are welcomed or good, but we ought not to view change in and of itself as a problem to be solved by medicine, as transhumanists seek to do by halting the regular progressions of aging. Women are perhaps most in tune with the ways in which the ebb and flow of bodily processes can be either destructive or generative.

Artist Christa Couture, for example, sought to celebrate her pregnancy in ways that resisted the common narratives of normalized pregnant women.[62] Couture's cosmesis floral covering on her prosthetic leg represented her body's transformation during pregnancy. "It literally decorated something that I'd be trying to hide," she writes. "It became something beautiful. Once I started to love my reflection with that accessory on, I was more easily able to love my reflection with it off."[63] Couture's pregnancy prosthesis highlighted her disability and helped her to love her body both with and without her assistive device. Once she was able to love her body, she was also able to love her transforming body. Just biotechnologies ought to be created with the understanding that the disabled body is desirable, generative, and transforming.

The dynamism of the body is not merely confined to this life. As Gregory of Nyssa describes in *The Life of Moses*, our journey toward

God in the afterlife might be also one of perpetual change—we continue to be transformed as we draw infinitely closer to the infinite God. Whereas many Christians believe they will receive permanent, perfect bodies in the resurrection, we might instead imagine our future bodies as continually changing as they approach God's infinite and ultimately unknowable self. Crip eschatology encourages us to *unknow* what we imagine as the perfect body.

Finally, eschatologically oriented biotechnologies should be *relational*. They ought to call forth deep relationships between people but also between user and device, animate and inanimate, and the human and the nonhuman world. Unlike the exoskeleton, which seems to want to dominate the disabled body, eschatological technologies ought to proceed from "a deep love for the disabled bodies,"[64] trying not to conquer them but to work with them in harmony.

Increasingly, physicians, designers, and prosthetic users come together to create bespoke wearables that incorporate clients' needs, desires, and aesthetics. Such prosthetics are meant to be shown off as artistic creations that suit the wearer's personality as well as enable their wearer to accomplish the tasks that make the wearer's life worthwhile. For example, a man identified as James worked with Summit ID to create a personalized prosthetic.[65] James was an avid motorcyclist before he lost his leg in an accident and wanted to regain that ability with his prosthetic. Rather than building a mass–produced prosthesis and then fit it to James, Summit ID used a 3–D printer to match the organic contours of James' body, while at the same time matching it to his beloved motorcycle. According to the company, their unique prosthetics are custom made, cheaper than most prosthetics, ecologically friendly, responsibly sourced, and often dishwasher safe.[66] Through their design process, the prosthesis is brought together with the individual, the individual with machine, and a bond is formed between the user and the designer, who each relinquish total control over the prosthesis in cooperation with one another. Seeing James, it is hard to tell where he ends and his motorcycle begins. This is not to suggest the kingdom of God is a place where our individual earthly desires are fulfilled but where creations are fitted more closely to their creator.

CONCLUSION

Crip technoscience can help expand the imagination of Christians who seek to describe what justice within the kingdom of God entails. Our common understanding of justice is often limited to our cultural understandings of ontology and the common good. In an ableist society, disability is seen as an inherently negative trait, and justice for the disabled has been associated with eliminating disability. It is no wonder, then, that many Christians imagine the kingdom of God as a place where disability is no more. The radical bodily and social transformation promised in the kingdom, however, may prompt us to reconceive our notions of justice and the place of disabled bodies within a just society.

Just prosthetics can evoke our kingdom imaginations by pointing toward their wearer's nonnormal embodiment. Rather than seeking to hide or overcome disability, prosthetics can be a site of rebellion against normativity. Of course, the refusal to wear a prosthesis can signal the same rejection of mandated normativity. Disability theologian Sharon Betcher, for example, refuses a prosthetic and instead chooses to display her missing limb more visibly by using crutches to move through the world. For Betcher, this choice is one of convenience and rebellion. She finds prosthetics uncomfortable and difficult to maneuver, but, just as importantly, she finds the prosthetic overly comfortable for those around her. She writes, "In my own experience, the day that I donned a prosthesis was the day that everyone else breathed a sigh of relief, and I lost my sense of humor."[67] For the disabled to simply exist as they are and resist the technological fix is a powerful symbol of the goodness of God's creation here and in the life to come.

For those who do use biotechnologies, however, they can signal a future reality wherein a diverse set of bodies will be celebrated. Certain technologies, even bioenhancements, stand out as signaling a kind of alternative future wherein disability remains, even while individual impairments are mitigated. Within certain crip biotechnologies, we see not a technological conquering of nature but a seamless fit between creators and creations. As we imagine a world in which all of God's creation is redeemed, restored, and reconciled, we ought to imagine that difference and disability remain.

Of course, such prosthetics are not isolated from our cultural depravities. Even prosthetics designed by people with disabilities may fall victim to the worst aspects of technocapitalism, which merely enhance one's personal control at the expense of their relationality. Prosthetics can reinforce as easily as they can challenge, as evidenced by the "Barbie" legs of athlete and fashion model Aimee Mullins, which she calls her "beautiful" legs. Bioenhancement technologies can reify in material bodies problematic gender constructions as well as class distinctions that were once only social constructions.[68] This is the thing about human beings: we are quick to pervert goodness; even the prosthetic invites technofetishism. This is, of course, the nature of sin, to distort the good. Christians must always be reminded that because of sin we will not bring about the kingdom through our own schemes, and, along with crip activists, we must resist the normalization of certain productive or beautiful bodies as well as the anti-relational values that often accompany them. The best we can do is point to the kingdom, perhaps even through our own technologies.

Notes

1   Julia Watts Belser, "Violence, Disability, and the Politics of Healing: The Inaugural Nancy Eiesland Endowment Lecture," *Journal of Disability & Religion* 19, no. 3 (2015): 177–97, 178.

2   Throughout this chapter, I will alternate between using the terms "people with disabilities" and "disabled people." The debates over first-person language vs. identity-first language are longstanding. As a disabled person, I prefer identity-first language but will seek to honor both perspectives by alternating my language.

3   The U.S. federal government typically funds around 27 percent of medical and health research and development in the United States. Research America, "U.S. Investments in Medical and Health Research and Development: 2013–2017," https://www.researchamerica.org/wp-content/uploads/2022/09/InvestmentReport2019_Fnl.pdf.

4   U.S. Department of Health and Human Services, "Social Determinants of Health," 2020, https://wayback.archive-it.org/5774/20220413203948/https://www.healthypeople.gov/2020/topics-objectives/topic/social-determinants-of-health.

5   T. Douglas, "Moral Enhancement," *Journal of Applied Philosophy* 25, no. 3 (2008): 228–45 (233).

6   Douglas, "Moral Enhancement," 233.

7   Nicholas Agar, "Moral Bioenhancement Is Dangerous," *Journal of Medical Ethics* 41, no. 4 (2015): 343–45; David Wasserman, "When Bad People Do Good Things: Will Moral Enhancement Make the World a Better Place?" *Journal of Medical Ethics* 40, no. 6 (2014): 374–75.

8   Plastic surgery in many countries is often covered by insurance when related to pathology (e.g., rhinoplasty for patients with respiratory problems or breast reconstruction surgery following mastectomy due to cancer), but such procedures are paid for because they are considered not enhancements but restoration of function or anatomical structure following disease.

9   Francis Fukuyama, "Transhumanism," *Foreign Policy* 144 (2009): 42–43, https://foreignpolicy.com/2009/10/23/transhumanism/.

10   "Transhumanist FAQ," website of Humanity+, https://www.humanityplus.org/transhumanist-faq.

11   "Transhumanist FAQ."

12   "Transhumanist FAQ."

13   Robert Sparrow, "Egalitarianism and Moral Bioenhancement," *American Journal of Bioethics* 14, no. 4 (2014): 20–28.

14   Alberto Giubilini and Francesca Minerva, "Enhancing Equality," *Journal of Medicine and Philosophy* 44, no. 3 (2019): 335–54 (344).

15   Giubilini and Minerva, "Enhancing Equality," 336.

16   Ron Amundson, "Disability, Ideology, and Quality of Life: A Bias in Biomedical Ethics," in *Quality of Life and Human Difference*, ed. David Wasserman, Jerome Bickenbach, and Robert Wachbroit (Cambridge: Cambridge University Press, 2005), 101–24 (103).

17   In his evangelical response to the genetic revolution, for example, John Jefferson Davis writes, "Creation as man experiences it, however, is not in its original state but fallen and imperfect and subject to 'bondage and decay.' Birth defects, including those of genetic origin, can be understood in relation to this fallenness of creation." Davis, "Christian Reflections on the Genetic Revolution," *Evangelical Review of Theology* 28, no. 1 (2004): 70.

18   Deborah B. Creamer, *Disability and Christian Theology: Embodied Limits and Constructive Possibilities* (New York: Oxford University Press, 2009).

19   Guy Kahane and Julian Savulescu, "The Welfarist Account of Disability," in *Disability and Disadvantage*, ed. Kimberley Brownlee and Adam Cureton (Oxford: Oxford University Press 2009), 14–53.

20   Giubilini and Minerva, "Enhancing Equality," 335–36.

21   Giubilini and Minerva, "Enhancing Equality," 344.

22   Giubilini and Minerva, "Enhancing Equality," 344.

23   "Great Jobs Great Lives: The 2014 Gallup-Purdue Index Report," Gallup, 2014, https://www.gallup.com/services/176768/2014-gallup-purdue -index-report.aspx.

24   The opportunity paradox actually holds that more opportunities do not lead to greater happiness. See Barry Schwartz, *The Paradox of Choice: Why More Is Less; How the Culture of Abundance Robs Us of Satisfaction* (New York: Harper Collins, 2005).

25   Elizabeth Barnes, *The Minority Body: A Theory of Disability* (Oxford: Oxford University Press 2016).

26   Stephen M. Campbell and Joseph A. Stramondo, "The Complicated Relationship of Disability and Well-Being," *Kennedy Institute of Ethics Journal* 27, no. 2 (2017): 151–84 (159).

27   Nancy Fraser, "Social Justice in the Age of Identity Politics: Redistribution, Recognition, and Participation," in *Redistribution or Recognition? A Political-Philosophical Exchange*, by Nancy Fraser and Alex Honneth (New York: Verso, 2003), 7–109.

28   Gary L. Albrecht and Patrick J. Devlieger, "The Disability Paradox," *Social Science and Medicine* 48, no. 8 (1999): 977–88.

29   Julian Savulescu, Melanie Hemsely, Ainsely Newson, and Bennet Foddy, "Behavioural Genetics: Why Eugenic Selection Is Preferable to Enhancement," *Journal of Applied Philosophy* 23, no. 2 (2006): 157–71.

30   Ingmar Persson and Julian Savulescu, "The Perils of Cognitive Enhancement and the Urgent Imperative to Enhance the Moral Character of Humanity," *Journal of Applied Philosophy* 25, no. 3 (2008): 162–77 (174).

31   Bostrom, "Human Genetic Enhancements," 493–506.

32   Carole Beighton and Jane Wills, "How Parents Describe the Positive Aspects of Parenting Their Child Who Has Intellectual Disabilities: A Systematic Review and Narrative Synthesis," *Journal of Applied Research in Intellectual Disability* 32 (2019): 1255–79.

33   Devan Stahl, *Disability's Challenge to Theology: Genes, Eugenics, and the Metaphysics of Modern Medicine* (Notre Dame: University of Notre Dame Press, 2022).

34   Rebecca F. Spurrier, *The Disabled Church: Human Difference and the Art of Communal Worship* (New York: Fordham, 2019), 3.

35   Alison Kafer, *Feminist, Queer, Crip* (Bloomington: Indiana University Press, 2013), 11.

36   Kafer, *Feminist*, 13. This distinction also falls within the Disability Justice Movement when compared with the Disability Rights Movement. "Disability Justice" as described by Patty Bernes and others notes that disability rights has focused exclusively on disability at the expense of other intersectional identities and creates hierarchies of disability

(those with mobility impairments at the top, with those with intel-lectual disabilities at the bottom). For more, see "What Is Disability Justice?" June 16, 2000, https://www.sinsinvalid.org/news-1/2020/6/16/what-is-disability-justice.

37   Donna J. Haraway, "A Cyborg Manifesto: Science, Technology and Socialist-Feminism in the Late Twentieth Century," in Donna J. Haraway, *Manifestly Haraway* (Minneapolis: University of Minnesota Press, 2016), https://doi.org/10.5749/minnesota/9780816650477.003.0001.

38   Alice Sheppard, "Staging Bodies, Performing Ramps: Cultural-Aesthetic Disability Technoscience," *Catalyst: Feminism, Theory, Technoscience* 5, no. 1 (2019): 1–12 (4).

39   Ray Kurzweil and Terry Grossman, *Transcend: Nine Steps to Living Well Forever* (New York: Rodale, 2010), 2.

40   Ray Kurzweil, *The Age of Spiritual Machines: When Computers Exceed Human Intelligence* (London: Penguin, 2000).

41   Methodius of Olympus believed human bodies would be melted down and reforged from the same material, such that their defects and damages would be eliminated. Similarly, Peter Lombard in *Four Books of Sentences* claims that resurrected bodies would be reconstituted with all their defects purged, "shining like the sun." He also argues that bodies would appear around thirty years old, but with every blemish removed. Many ancient and medieval theologians contended that res-urrected bodies would be thirty or thirty-three years old (depending on when they believed Jesus died)—and *very* able-bodied—perhaps even male. This contrasts strongly with Gregory of Nyssa's rumination on the resurrection, in which he writes, "If our bodies are to live again in every respect the same as before, this thing that we are expect-ing is simply a calamity; whereas if they are not the same, the per-son raised up will be another than he who died"—to which Macrina responds that the resurrection is a mystery. Gregory of Nyssa, *On the Soul and the Resurrection*, trans. William Moore and Henry Austin Wil-son, in *Nicene and Post-Nicene Fathers: Second Series*, vol. 5, ed. Philip Schaff and Henry Wace (Buffalo, N.Y.: Christian Literature Publishing, 1893). Revised and edited for New Advent by Kevin Knight: http://www.newadvent.org/fathers/2915.htm.

42   Nancy L. Eiesland, *The Disabled God: Toward a Liberatory Theology of Disability* (Nashville: Abingdon, 1994), 89–105.

43   See Creamer, *Disability*; and Thomas E. Reynolds, *Vulnerable Com-munion: A Theology of Disability and Hospitality* (Grand Rapids: Brazos, 2008).

44   Amos Yong, *Theology and Down Syndrome: Reimagining Disability in Later Modernity* (Waco, Tex.: Baylor University Press, 2007), 282.

45 Richard Cross, "Duns Scotus on Disability: Teleology, Divine Willing, and Pure Nature," *Theological Studies* 78, no. 1 (2017): 72–95.

46 Cross, "Duns Scotus," 94.

47 Sharon Betcher, "Putting My Foot (Prosthesis, Crutches, Phantom) Down: Considering Technology as Transcendence in the Writings of Donna Haraway," *Women's Studies Quarterly* 29, nos. 3/4 (2001): 49.

48 Ashraf Gorgey, "Robotic Exoskeletons: The Current Pros and Cons," *World Journal of Orthopedics* 9, no. 9 (2018): 112–19 (113).

49 Jathan Sadowski, "Exoskeletons in a Disabilities Context: The Need for Social and Ethical Research," *Journal of Responsible Innovation* 1, no. 2 (2014): 214–19.

50 Jean Thilmany, "Exoskeletons for Construction Workers Are Marching On-Site," *Constructible*, February 27, 2019, https://constructible .trimble.com/construction-industry/exoskeletons-for-construction -workers-are-marching-on-site.

51 Esko Bionics (@Esko Bionics), "Sometimes, care lives in an empty wheelchair," Twitter, September 26, 2016, https://twitter.com/ eksobionics/status/1177277981393346563.

52 "Esko Bionics," CUNY Assistive Technology Services, accessed September 13, 2021, http://cats.cuny.edu/ekso-bionics/.

53 Alison Kafer, "Crip Kin, Manifesting," *Catalyst: Feminism, Theory, Technoscience* 5, no. 1 (2019): 1–37 (11).

54 Steven Ashley, "Robotic Exoskeletons Are Changing Lives in Surprising Ways," *NBC News*, February 21, 2017, https://www.nbcnews.com/mach/ innovation/robotic-exoskeletons-are-changing-lives-surprising -ways-n722676.

55 "A Robotic Exoskeleton Works Miracles," *MIT Technology Review*, May 20, 2011, https://www.technologyreview.com/2011/05/20/194588/a-robotic -exoskeleton-works-miracles/.

56 Zolton Istvan, "In the Transhumanist Age, We Should Be Repairing Disabilities, Not Sidewalks," *Vice News*, April 3, 2015, https://www.vice .com/en_us/article/4x3pdm/in-the-transhumanist-age-we-should -be-repairing-disabilities-not-sidewalks.

57 Istvan, "Transhumanist Age."

58 "White House Fashion Show Celebrating Inclusive Design, Assistive Technology, and Prosthetics," YouTube video, 13:31, posted by the Obama White House, September 15, 2016, https://www.youtube.com/ watch?v=tXytHqOe-N8.

59 Andrea Shea, "Remembering Lisa Bufano, a Dancer Who Found Beauty in Amputation," *WBR News*, December 24, 2013, https://www.wbur.org/ artery/2013/12/24/lisa-bufano-remembrance.

60   Sonsherée Giles, "One Breath Is an Ocean for a Wooden Heart,"http://www.sonsheree.com/project/one-breath-ocean-wooden-heart.

61   Rosemarie Garland Thomson, *Extraordinary Bodies: Figuring Physical Disability in American Culture and Literature* (New York: Columbia University Press, 1997), 8.

62   "About," website of Christa Couture, http://christacouture.com/about/.

63   Christa Couture, "That Time I Went Viral—For My Pregnancy Photos," website of Christa Couture, June 27, 2018, http://christacouture.com/that-time-i-went-viral-for-my-pregnancy-photos/.

64   Kafer, *Feminist*, 13.

65   "Scott Summit Brings Individuality to Prosthetic Leg Fairings with 3D Technology," website of 3D Systems, accessed July 6, 2023, https://www.3dsystems.com/customer-stories/scott-summit-puts-personal-design-and-manufacturing-prosthetic-leg-fairings.

66   Scott Summit, "Beautiful Artificial Limbs," November 2011, TEDxCambridge, video, 10:55, https://www.ted.com/talks/scott_summit_beautiful_artificial_limbs/transcript?language=en.

67   Betcher, "Putting My Foot," 42.

68   Chris Hables Gray and Steven Mentor, "The Cyborg Body Politic and the New World Order," in *Prosthetic Territories: Politics and Hypertechnologies*, ed. Gabriel Brahm Jr. and Mark Driscoll (Boulder, Colo.: Westview, 1995), 204–17, 245, n. 7.

EPILOGUE
Enhancing Bodies: From What to What?
John Swinton

It is difficult to know what I can say that has not already been said in the fascinating and important essays that have been presented in this volume. The richness, diversity, and depth of the essays presented here is impressive. The volume as a whole sets the tone for a series of new, innovative, and hopefully transformative conversations around an issue that is fundamentally important in relation to the kind of church we are, the type of society we want for the future, and ultimately what it means to be human in an imperfect world. As someone who has spent many years working alongside people living with disabilities and thinking through the theological implications of lives that are perceived to be different, the issue of normality and therapeutic change has always been on my horizon. What it means to be normal is complex. Who decides what is normal is deeply political. Why we desire to be normal in the ways that we do is a complex mishmash of societal pressure, personal desire, and, often, theological misunderstanding. Who can actually afford to make the changes necessary to achieve societal and personal norms and desires is a matter of economics and social justice. Normality is not only a myth; it is a battlefield!

Bioenhancement speaks to the question of normality in important ways. At heart, bioenhancement relates to the augmentation of human bodies or human capacities, brought about through some kind of biological manipulation. There is an assumed norm within this practice that functions at a cultural/societal level and at a personal level. The desire may be to achieve that norm, or to surpass it. It is not insignificant that the aim is rarely, if ever, to move someone *below* the assumed cultural norm in relation to any physical or psychological state. By definition, bioenhancement ignores, moves away from, and potentially downgrades those people who sit below or outside of the assumed norm. If I think having super eyesight is a desirable goal, I have to assume that having poor eyesight or being blind is less desirable. When one marks out an experience as less desirable or even undesirable, it is a small step to mark out a person or a group of people as undesirable. While this may not be an overt goal of bioenhancement, it is clearly a significant implication.

At the cultural and societal levels, the nature and outcome of bioenhancement is shaped and formed by desires and expectations that emerge from the particular contexts that create the technology necessary for the enhancement. It is therefore not surprising that, in a rapidly secularizing Western context, something like death should be seen as a primary focus of attention. In a world that has lost the narratives of providence, sanctification, resurrection, and life after death, one would expect a primary focus to be on avoiding death and those things that remind us of our mortality. It is also not surprising, as the essays in this volume have clearly shown, that the criteria for what should be enhanced will be determined by the wealthy, the powerful, and those who think that they understand the nature of beauty and the good life. Those on the margins are inevitably excluded and implicitly or explicitly urged to acknowledge that their own beauty is not in fact beautiful and that, if they can afford it, they should conform their bodies to the majority expectation. There is a lot at stake in this conversation, and these practices and the essayists in this volume have drawn this out clearly. In this closing reflection, I want to offer some brief reflections on theology and the body, which I hope will mingle well with the wisdom presented by others.

What Did Adam Look Like? What Does the Genesis Account of Creation Tell Us about Perceptions of Normality?

I am fascinated by the criteria that people use in relation to what they think should be enhanced by human biotechnology. If they are to develop their theological reflection authentically, it is important that Christians are clear about what they think a body should look like and what it is for. The field of disability theology has unsettled Christian assumptions about what is and what is not normal and what it might mean to change people from one way of being in the world to another. One of the central concerns that people have in relation to, for example, the healing ministry is that healing very quickly becomes a mode of normalization and divine bioenhancement if we are not theologically sensitive to some key issues. One of the things that Scripture does well is to raise our consciousness to issues that we easily overlook. Reflection on Scripture transforms our minds (Rom 12:2) and raises our consciousness to different aspects of creation that cannot be seen without its illumination.[1] When this happens, change happens.

It is interesting to note that the Genesis accounts of creation do not refer to creation as being perfect. It is very good, but perfection is something that only comes with the descent of the new Jerusalem in the book of Revelation (Rev 21). David Ferguson puts it this way:

> Creation is imperfect and incomplete. The making of the world is only the first of God's works. As the beginning of a history, it sets in motion a narrative that has a focal point in the coming of Jesus. The ordering of the Christian canon itself suggests a pattern of promise and fulfilment. God's creative work is ongoing throughout the history of Israel and the church, even embracing resistance and struggle in its dealing with people and natural forces.[2]

We are on a journey toward *God's* understanding of perfection. The question is, *what does that perfection actually look like?* The answer is, of course, it looks like Jesus (Heb 5:9)! It is as we obey Jesus, love God, and come to know God that we discover the nature of divine perfection (1 John 2:5). We look to Jesus for our image of perfection. This seems straightforward. However, when one asks the question of exactly what Jesus looks like, things become complicated.

Alongside of the lack of perfection in creation and the divine movement toward God's ideal of perfection, we also note that the first humans were also not perfect or somehow clothed in God's glory. Again, this seems obvious. However, it has not always been obvious within the tradition. As Joel Estes points out:

> Nothing in Genesis 2 or in the history of its interpretation suggests that the first humans were anything other than fully "abled" individuals. Indeed, in the history of exegesis and art they are not only perfect humans but, in some cases, depicted as super-human. In numerous Rabbinic texts, for example, Adam's body is gigantic, embodies all of the physical perfections of Israel's historic heroes, and displays a splendor that eclipses even the sun.[3]

However, as Talitha Cooreman-Guittin points out, such tradition is flawed:

> There is no mention of humankind being pure or unblemished or perfect neither in Gen 1 nor in Gen 2–3. Paul Ricoeur put it this way: "All the speculations about the supernatural perfection of Adam before the fall are adventitious arrangements that profoundly alter the original meaning, naïve and crude; they tend to make Adam superior and therefore foreign to our condition, and thereby reduce the Adamic myth to a genesis of man from primordial superhumanity."[4]

This is an important observation. If everything is imperfect, then rather than attempting to single out oneself or other people as imperfect and in need of enhancement, perhaps a better strategy might be to love everything within creation (including ourselves) in the way that God loves creation. Creation stands as a statement that God loves diversity and not homogeneity. The only beauty that counts is the beauty that God sees in us.

There is, however, a problem here. In the same way as the question of what Jesus looks like is unanswerable, so the question of the nature of God's idea of beauty is not obvious to fallen human beings. To the question, *What does God's idea of beauty and perfection actually look like?* our truthful answer must be that *we really do not know.* Returning to the Genesis account of creation, it is important to notice that nowhere in the accounts are we told what Adam looked like. We do not know how tall he was, how small he was, how many arms he had, how fit he was, how scarred he was, how intelligent he was; we do not know whether he would have lived forever if he had not sinned or whether he aged in the same way as we do. We can guess and argue about it, but Scripture simply does not give us such information. It is therefore difficult to work out what kinds of bioenhancement we might support in relation to moving human bodies and minds toward God's ideal of beauty and perfection.

The observation that Scripture does not inform us or our original biological form is important for the discussion around bioenhancement. It means that our assumptions about normality and beauty and our desire to enhance our bodies or our minds are inevitably *projections*: imaginative creations based on the information that we have available to us at any moment in time, context, and history. If *I* imagine Adam as embodying *my* ideas of what a perfect human being is, then *I* will assume that anything that does not meet *my* assumed criterion requires adjustment. This projected way of looking at the world easily spills into our theological assumptions, expectations, and practices. I might, for example, assume that that which is not pleasing or beautiful to me or my community is the consequence of the fall and as such requires spiritual bioenhancement (healing). This, sadly, is a not uncommon response to disability. One of the problems with the church's healing ministry is that it often assumes that both healer and the one who desires healing know what kind of enhancement they need in order to be "normal." When we begin to think in this way, it is those on the margins who become the object of divine bioenhancement with obvious negative consequences. Rather than thinking through the implications and living into the mystery of Genesis 2, the temptation is to race toward Genesis 3. Projecting the things that human beings desire onto people and persuading them (and yourself) that they are the things that God wants is a pretty neat definition of sin.

Projection functions in both church and society to construct norms that are inevitably dangerous for people considered "abnormal," be that because of disability, race, sex, or whatever. Projected aesthetics and normate expectations become a battleground that is more political than biblical, more sociological than theological, more oppressive than liberating. As we consider issues around normality and what needs to be enhanced and why, we would be wise to spend a little time dwelling in the implications of Genesis 2 and the need to think about what it might mean to be reflexive and project faithfully (for project we will).

WHICH BODY SHOULD WE ENHANCE? THE LIVED BODY AND THE MATERIAL BODY

The Genesis account of creation provides us with useful insights into how and why we construct the norms that underpin the desire to enhance our bodies. But there is another issue around bodies that is not foregrounded in the various discussions around bioenhancement—that is, *what do we mean when we are thinking about "the body"?* Bioenhancement relates to the physical manipulation of the body. As such, those who engage with such practices tend to be deeply materialistic in terms of what they think the body is, what it is for, what it should look like, and how it should function. There is, however, an aspect of bodily life that is not generally reflected on in these kinds of conversation. Within the philosophical field of phenomenology, a distinction is made between the *material* body and the *lived* body.[5] The material body is the physicality of our being: that which provides us with the physical basis for our existence. The material body grounds us in the world and enables the possibility of awareness, identity, selfhood, meaningful life, and so forth. The material body is the locus of manipulations for those engaging in bioenhancement. The material body is also a locus for our spiritual life and our connectedness with God and others. In the Genesis account of creation, God creates Adam out of the dust (Gen 2:7). God blows God's *ruach* into Adam, and he becomes a person. Human beings are made from dust and return to dust. As Augustine puts it in his *City of God*, human beings are *terra animata*: animated dust.[6] There is no indication here of a separate dimension that we might call the soul. Body, mind, soul is inextricably interconnected. What happens in one realm impacts upon all realms. We are our bodies as we are our souls. The material body is thus seen to be both soulful and relational. *Bioenhancement is inevitably a matter of the soul*. If biotechnologies are not to become anything more than the manifestation of self-adoration wherein the body becomes a vehicle for personal gratification, we need to bear in mind that our bodies are a soulful temple within which the Holy Spirit dwells and through which the ongoing mission of God is manifested (1 Cor 6:9). This is important. Manipulating bodies for purposes other than God's may bring a degree of temporal happiness and security about the future (I do not have to die anymore!), but, in overlooking the soulfulness of the body, bioenhancement can very easily become a source of idolatry. As well as being important for theological ethics, there is a crucial missiological dimension to this aspect of the conversation that is not always noted.

This missiological dimension is brought out in an interesting way via the experience of Paul in 2 Corinthians 12:8–10:

> Three times I pleaded with the Lord to take it away from me. But he said to me, "My grace is sufficient for you, for my power is made perfect in weakness." Therefore I will boast all the more gladly about my weaknesses, so that Christ's power may rest on me. That is why, for Christ's sake, I delight in weaknesses, in insults, in hardships, in persecutions, in difficulties. For when I am weak, then I am strong. (NIV)

Paul, the greatest missionary of all time, prays to God to be healed, and God says no. Instead, Paul discovers that his strength is to be found in the thing that he wanted to change. There is something powerful here. A profound danger with bioenhancement is that we end up "enhancing" and changing the very things that God wants to use in his mission of reconciliation in, to, and for the world. What *we* might think are wonderful changes are not necessarily what God sees as wonderful changes. Recognizing the soulfulness of bodies and the vocational nature of human beings is important.

The Lived Body

Alongside the material body (not apart from it), phenomenologists talk about the *lived body*. The idea of the lived body relates to the ways in which the material body experiences the world as it moves through it. The lived body has to do with a person's lived relationship toward and with the world. The lived body is the acting, perceiving subject, accessed by way of subjective self-reflection. The lived body occurs or emerges as we move through the world. It is here that we discover our identity; our place in the world; the meaning and purpose of our lives and the kinds of things that enhance or detract from our lived goals. Conversations around bioenhancement need to take material bodies seriously, but they also need to think about the moral goals of such bodies and what happens when enhanced bodies are lived.

PAUL, THE BODY, AND BIOENHANCEMENT

In concluding this reflection, it will be helpful to turn to Paul's theology of the body, which has important implications for our developing understanding of the soulful and lived dimensions of bioenhancement. In her important paper "Bodies, Agency, and the Relational Self: A Pauline Approach to the Goals and Use of Psychiatric Drugs,"[7] New Testament scholar Susan Eastman discusses the implications of Paul's theology of the body for the use of psychopharmacology. Her argument around medication resonates in important ways with the conversation being laid out in this chapter. For Paul, Eastman argues, *participation* is central to understanding the body:

> Paul views the body as a mode of participation in larger relational matrices in both vulnerable and vital ways. He thus sees the self as constituted relationally rather than as fundamentally isolated and self-determining. Such an understanding of personhood yields an account of human agency as co-constituted and freedom as interpersonally mediated and sustained.[8]

Counter to the idea that we are discrete individuals who reside within our own bodies quite apart from the bodies of others, Paul informs us that we are who we are, and we do what we do as we participate with others in outward spirals of relationality. Our material bodies are necessary, but they are not sufficient. They need to be lived in particular ways. The body is not an enclosed unit but rather a relational entity that constantly seeks to bridge the gap between itself and the bodies of others:

> It is as if physical bodies were bridges rather than barriers, making human creatures into participatory beings, not autonomous, not isolated, but connected to larger "bodies."[9]

The self emerges from participation in ever-expanding relational matrices. It is as we participate in relationships with others that we discover ourselves. In this understanding we are both independent and dependent:

We are interdependent selves, not fully absorbed into a communal identity, but also never fully self-reliant and self-contained. From a Pauline perspective on human freedom, agency, and well-being, therefore, the goal is always life-giving connection, not discrete, self-directed, and self-sufficient individualism. Indeed, from Paul's perspective, the claim to be completely self-sufficient, free-standing, isolated persons would be a lethal delusion.[10]

Embodiment is fundamental to personhood now and also in the life to come:

What is sown is perishable, what is raised is imperishable. It is sown in dishonor, it is raised in glory. It is sown in weakness, it is raised in power. It is sown a physical body, it is raised a spiritual. If there is a physical body, there is also a spiritual body. (1 Cor 15:42–44, NRSV)

There can be no separation between our personhood and our physical, embodied existence: "Our selfhood is grounded and sustained by relational bonds."[11]

Necessary Vulnerability

For Paul, bodies are intended to exist "in the mode of belonging."[12] We belong to others and ultimately to God. Belonging in this mode means that human beings are inevitably and necessarily profoundly vulnerable. The social matrix that persons are involved with can be healthy and healing, but it can also be deeply destructive. The ways in which we configure our relationships will determine whether we live healthily or destructively:

When the relational matrix to which individuals belong is life-giving and communicates grace, such belonging does not negate individuality; in fact, it creates it, as Paul's words, "individually members of the Body of Christ," suggest. Paul does not convey a competitive account of the relationship between divine and human agents in which the more God acts, the less humans act. To the contrary, God's action strengthens and amplifies human action. The iteration of such noncompetitive agencies in human interactions is as a kind of allied agency; our capacities to know, decide, and act in effective ways are co-constituted in relationship with God and other people.[13]

This view of the body moves us away from both materialism and dualism. The material dimensions of our body are important. But so also is the lived body as it reaches out and relates to the world. Here we discover the fullness of persons. Paul's thinking also moves us away from dualism. There is no room for a disembodied understanding of the mind or the self: "To be a mind without a body would be, in Paul's language, to be 'naked' or 'unclothed' (2 Cor. 5:2–4)."[14] What we do with our bodies and what we do with our minds are not separate things. They are deeply interlinked, with what occurs in one impacting on the other and vice versa.

THE MORAL GOAL OF BIOENHANCEMENT

These very brief reflections on Pauline perspectives on personhood and the body show the centrality of the body as the ground of our personhood and the ways in which the body is foundationally relational and participatory. With this in mind, it seems clear that the proper goal of bioenhancement is not simply to bring about personal changes that make people happier or more conformed to a cultural or personal norm. Rather, the moral goal of bioenhancement should be to remove barriers that prevent the kinds of relationships and human connections that hold us in our personhood. Viewed as a communal practice with a relational goal, we can see that there may be times and issues where bioenhancement can be a faithful practice. Rather than being simply a technical, biologically oriented action, bioenhancement can be seen as a relational process that takes seriously the soulfulness of the material body and the deep relationality of the lived body and that seeks to help move a person toward the kind of identity, agency, and relationship that God desires. Bioenhancement, faithfully practiced, allows the development of "life giving connection rather than self-directed, self sufficient individualism."[15]

Enhancing Faithfully

In the light of what we have discussed thus far, the questions asked by those involved with bioenhancement cannot simply be "Does this procedure work?" if the definition of what "work" means is not clear. Does "work" mean fixing and mending an individual? Does "work" mean moving away from the fear of death? Does "work" mean conforming to a cultural or personal norm? Does "work" mean making life happier, more productive for the individual? Does "work" mean making life easier for individuals and families? Does "work" mean making life easier for society? Or does "work" mean helping people to renegotiate their relational connectedness in ways that bring about life in all of its fullness? While all of these aspects of "work" may be important, the latter seems to be the overarching priority that gives the other forms of "work" their telos and goal. There are four questions that we might want to bear in mind in the light of the arguments of this paper:

(1) In what sense does this procedure facilitate a person's movement into relationship with God, self, and others?

(2) For whose benefit is this procedure administered (the individual, society, etc.)?

(3) What will the person gain through this procedure?

(4) What will a person lose if this procedure is administered?

Questions such as these help us to remember the lived body, take seriously the soulfulness of the material body, and use our technology to enable the maintenance and development of the personhood of individuals and communities.

In this essay I have tried to lay down some theological reflections that can add to the great wisdom of the essays presented in this book. There is much more that can be said, but I suspect that if people take seriously the wisdom presented in this book, the world might just be a better place for all of us together.

NOTES

1 St. Augustine describes illumination in this way: "When we lift up our eyes to the scriptures, because the scriptures have been provided by human beings, we are lifting up our eyes to the mountains from where help will come to us. Even so, because those who wrote the scriptures were human beings, they were not shining on their own, but he was the true light who illumines everyone coming into this world (John 1:9)."

2 David Fergusson, *Creation* (Grand Rapids: Eerdmans, 2014), 9.

3 Joel Estes, "Imperfection in Paradise: Reading Genesis 2 through the Lens of Disability and a Theology of Limits," *Horizons in Biblical Theology* 38 (2016): 10.

244 | John Swinton

4   Talitha Cooreman-Guittin, "Could Adam and Eve Have Been Dis-
     abled? Images of Creation in Catholic Religious Education Textbooks
     in France," *Journal of Disability & Religion* 22, no. 1 (2018): 91.

5   Maren Wehrle, "Being a Body and Having a Body: The Twofold Tem-
     porality of Embodied Intentionality," *Phenomenology and the Cogni-
     tive Sciences* 19 (2020): 499–521; Gunn Engelsrud, "The Lived Body as
     Experience and Perspective: Methodological Challenges," *Qualitative
     Research* 5, no. 3 (2005): 267–84.

6   Gilbert Meilaender, "*Terra Es Animata* on Having a Life," *Hastings Center
     Report* 23, no. 4 (1993): 25–32.

7   Susan G. Eastman, "Bodies, Agency, and the Relational Self: A Pau-
     line Approach to the Goals and Use of Psychiatric Drugs," *Christian
     Bioethics: Non-ecumenical Studies in Medical Morality* 24, no. 3 (2018):
     288–301.

8   Eastman, "Bodies," 288.

9   Eastman, "Bodies," 292.

10   Eastman, "Bodies," 290–91.

11   Eastman, "Bodies," 293.

12   Eastman, "Bodies," 299.

13   Eastman, "Bodies," 293.

14   Eastman, "Bodies," 291.

15   Eastman, "Bodies," 291.